Dirty Dairy

Dirty Dairy

The Biological, Hormonal, & Neurological Consequences of Dairy Consumption

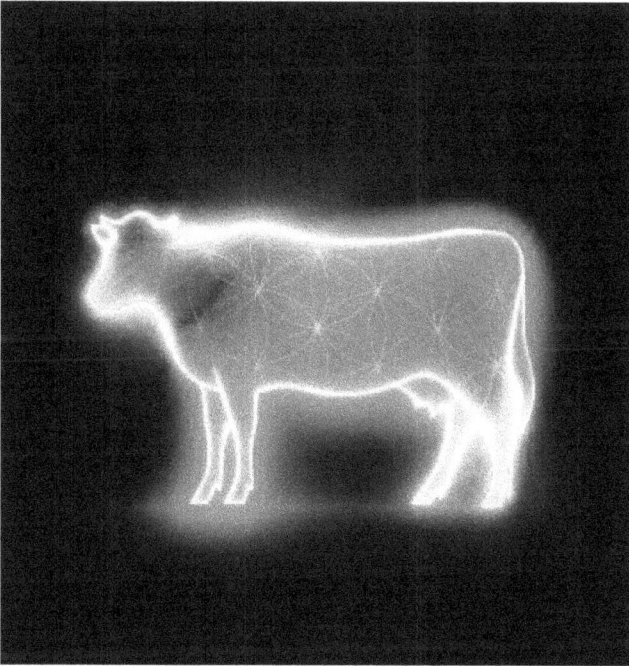

How Butter, Cheese, Ghee, Milk & Whey Disrupt Human Biology

Jesse J. Jacoby &
Anthony Lowther

Soulspire Publishing
Truckee, CA, 96161

ISBN: 978-1-968660-35-2
Library of Congress Control Number: 2012921011
Dewey CIP: 641.563   **OCLC:** 213839254

Cover art, font, and layout are all original art by: Abdul Rehman

Wholesalers to book trade: Nelson's Books and Ingram
Available through Amazon.com, BarnesAndNoble.com

Dedication

To every person who has ever questioned the narrative on their plate, felt the quiet whisper of their body asking for something cleaner, or sensed that the truth has always been simpler than the stories we were told.

To the animals whose suffering seeded our awakening. Your lives were not in vain. May this work help end the cycle that never should have begun.

To Earth, the great mother who never stops offering what heals, we dedicate this book to the return of clarity, compassion, and nourishment that honors all life.

Finally, to future generations, may the world you inherit be lighter, clearer, and free from the burdens we chose to release.

Acknowledgments

This book was born from thousands of pages of research, hundreds of lived experiments, and a shared commitment to uncovering what our physiology has been trying to tell us all along.

To the scientists, researchers, and pioneers who challenge convention with evidence and courage. Your work laid the foundation for this truth.

To the global community of plant-based physicians, integrative practitioners, and nutritional visionaries. Thank you for holding the line when the world was not yet ready to listen.

To our families, who supported our obsessions with data, our endless drafts, and our pursuit of purity. Your love made this book possible.

To the readers, for your willingness to question, examine, and evolve. Your openness is the spark that transforms culture.

To every animal whose story lives silently behind the dairy and meat industries. Your suffering has shaped our resolve. This book is part of our vow to end the dominion.

Finally, to each other, for the conversations, the science, and the shared vision of a world where nourishment means no being must pay the price.

The Research Trail

Introduction: The White Lie

White has always carried a sacred symbolism as the color of purity, divinity, and renewal. In the modern diet, however, there is a white that masquerades as innocence. The frothing swirl of milk, sheen of butter, and seduction of melted cheese stretching across a slice of bread are emblems of comfort, nostalgia, and supposed nourishment. Beneath their smooth surface, however, lies a biological betrayal.

The dairy industry has woven one of the most successful illusions in human history. We were told that milk *"does a body good,"* strengthens bones, grows children, and sustains vitality. Biology, chemistry, and cellular intelligence tell a very different story. Beneath the marketing gloss, dairy is not a food of life but a *signal of confusion* in the human body that hijacks hormones, dulls cellular communication, congests the lymphatic rivers, and veils our vitality beneath layers of mucosal decay.

Milk was meant for calves. This is a growth fluid perfectly engineered to transform a sixty-pound newborn into a 600-pound mammal in months. Human biology was never designed to endure the growth factors, hormones, and proteins embedded within bovine milk. Each sip is a whisper of foreign command and genetic message written in cow's code, entering the temple of human flesh.

At the molecular level, milk is not gentle. The casein protein fraction breaks down into casomorphins. These opioid peptides bind to receptors in the brain, sedating awareness and fostering addiction. Cheese is biochemically engineered for dependency. Concentrated casein is wrapped in saturated fat, delivering dopamine spikes that mirror the pathways of narcotics. This is why cheese cravings resist reason. The tongue is fooled by the brain's pleasure chemistry while the blood thickens and bowels slow.

Casein is a protein used in industrial glue because of the stickiness. When digested, this glue floods the bloodstream with inflammatory residues that promote tumor growth, a connection first illuminated by Dr. T. Colin Campbell in *The China Study*. Casein amplifies IGF-1 (Insulin-Like Growth Factor 1), the hormone that accelerates cellular proliferation. This is a process beneficial only for infant growth or cancer. The same biochemical cascade that tells a calf to grow is now telling human tumors to expand.

The fat molecules in dairy carry their own burden. Through homogenization, fat globules are mechanically shattered and oxidized, allowing a reactive enzyme known as xanthine oxidase to slip through intestinal walls and scar arterial linings. Through pasteurization, enzymes and beneficial bacteria are annihilated, transforming a living liquid into a sterile sludge that ferments into acid-forming byproducts. Even so-called *"raw"* or *"grass-fed"* milk cannot escape the nature that this remains a breeding ground for acid-forming bacteria and endotoxins, taxing the immune system and corroding inner equilibrium. The chyle, that sacred milky fluid which builds our blood, becomes heavy, stagnant, and unworthy of constructing life's finer tissues after ingesting dairy.

Each glass of milk carries a hormonal storm of estrogen, progesterone, cortisol, and bovine growth hormones that were never meant to enter the human endocrine orchestra. In the bloodstream, they disrupt ovulation, fuel acne, feed fibroids, and burden the prostate. For men, they silence testosterone, and for women, they distort cycles of creation. The body's chemistry becomes enslaved to an alien rhythm and the pulse of another species.

Meanwhile, at the microscopic frontier, dairy fosters inflammation in the gut. Casein binds with gliadin, the wheat protein that constructs gluten, forming a complex that the immune system mistakes for an invader. The intestinal lining that is delicate, electric, and alive then begins to tear. Tight junctions loosen. Lipopolysaccharides (LPS), which are bacterial fragments from dairy fermentation, then leak into the bloodstream, igniting systemic fire. This *"leaky gut"* is the genesis of autoimmune chaos, mood disorders, and the slow erosion of vitality.

The story of milk is not one of nourishment, but of confusion. We learn of a species consuming another species' growth fluid, expecting vitality but inheriting stagnation. The irony is cosmic in that we drink milk to become strong, yet this substance saps strength. We seek comfort, yet drinking milk from other species clogs the body's rivers of renewal.

We live in a time where the purity of white must be reclaimed, not in color, but in consciousness. True purity arises when the fluids of the body run clear, lymph moves freely, and blood carries light instead of sludge. This book is more than a condemnation of dairy but is a biological exorcism of a cultural addiction. This is our call to remember what true nourishment feels like. This is a reminder that we can have clean breath, bright eyes, and cells that sing.

Dairy is a frequency, not a food, and when the body is tuned to truth, the resonance of that frequency is revealed as a distortion in the symphony of life.

Chapter 1: Not Food for Humans

When Nourishment Becomes Noise

There is a sacred design written into every species, and the milk of each mother is a code for her young. This is the first language of life and a biochemical lullaby sung from one body to another. In that milk is the blueprint for immunity, growth, and adaptation.

This design is precise and non-transferable. To drink another species' milk is to steal instructions from a foreign script, forcing the human body to translate what was never written for us.

The Language of Milk

Cow's milk contains more than sixty active hormones, hundreds of distinct proteins foreign to human tissue, and a molecular ratio designed to transform a sixty-pound calf into a 600-pound cow in less than a year. Dairy is not encoded with any instructions to refine the neural complexity of a human being.

The casein-to-whey ratio (80: 20) contrasts sharply with the (40: 60) of human milk. That imbalance alone alters digestion, kidney load, and hormonal signaling. Once ingested, bovine proteins such as casein, β-lactoglobulin, bovine serum albumin, and immunoglobulins reach the intestinal lining intact. Because they are xenogenic (foreign to the human proteome), they can cross a compromised gut barrier and enter circulation. There they trigger confusion at the cellular level, provoking inflammatory cascades and antibody formation.

This is the beginning of xenogenic integration, which is the forced merging of animal molecules into human biochemistry. Our intelligent and selective cell membranes attempt to interpret these invaders, but their geometry and receptor affinities do not match. The result is biochemical interference that is expressed through distorted signaling, oxidative stress, and accelerated telomere shortening. Telomere length is the cellular clock of aging.

Over time, the immune system begins mistaking the body's own tissues for these invaders. This is a process called molecular mimicry, and is the spark behind many autoimmune syndromes, including Hashimoto's thyroiditis, rheumatoid arthritis, lupus, and type 1 diabetes. What we call *"aging"* is often the slow corrosion of clarity as the immune system fights ghosts of foreign code.

Milk as a Growth Signal

Milk is a growth message, and the creamy swirl carries IGF-1 (Insulin-Like Growth Factor 1), estrogen, progesterone, and bovine growth hormone, all engineered to multiply cells at rapid speed. In a calf, this is sacred engineering. In an adult human, this becomes biochemical chaos and is expressed in the experience of acne, cystic inflammation, fibroids, PCOS, and even cancerous proliferation tracing back to these unchecked growth signals.

The same hormone that builds bone in a calf accelerates tumor formation in humans. The same fluid that produces muscle mass in livestock thickens the human waistline with edema and stored fat.

Calcium & the Great Nutrient Illusion

The dairy industry's proudest myth claims that milk *"builds strong bones."* Yet nations with the highest milk intake, being the U.S., Finland, and Sweden suffer the highest fracture rates. The paradox is chemical.

Dairy protein, rich in sulfur-containing amino acids, metabolizes into sulfuric acid. To maintain blood pH, the body leaches calcium phosphate from bone to buffer that acid. Thus, dairy gives calcium with one hand and steals calcium with the other.

True bone integrity arises from alkaline minerals that include magnesium, boron, silica, and plant-based calcium from sesame, kale, amaranth, figs, and leafy greens. These form flexible collagen scaffolds. Calcium, stripped of plant cofactors, creates brittleness instead of strength.

Lactase Persistence: A Mutation, Not a Milestone

Roughly sixty-five percent of adults worldwide lose the enzyme lactase after weaning. A minority carry a mutation allowing continued lactose digestion. This is known as lactase persistence. A trait born from famine survival, not superior evolution.

To keep drinking milk beyond infancy is to prolong biochemical childhood. When undigested lactose ferments in the colon, this yields hydrogen gas, lactic acid, and endotoxins, producing bloating, acidosis, and immune activation. The body's *"intolerance"* is wisdom, saying, *this does not belong here.*

Species-Specific Design

Each mammal's milk mirrors their destiny:

• Seal milk contains fifty percent fat for Arctic insulation.

• Giraffe milk is dense with minerals from acacia foliage.

• Elephant milk carries immune peptides that sustain seven-decade longevity.

• Human milk is low in protein, high in glucose, and rich in antibodies, crafted for brain growth and immune sophistication.

To ingest cow's milk is to download the blueprint of another species bred for bulk, not consciousness. The biochemical message is *"Grow fast, store fat, multiply cells."* Human milk whispers *"Refine, connect, awaken."* When we drink milk meant for calves, we trade refinement for rapidity, and awareness for accumulation.

Digestive Disarray and Mucosal Memory

The human digestive tract thrives on enzymatic, fiber-rich foods that leave no residue. Dairy behaves differently as casein curds adhere to the intestinal villi. These finger-like absorptive hairs feed the bloodstream.

This coating becomes a mucoprotein film, reducing nutrient uptake and dulling electro-chemical signaling between cells. The lymphatic system thickens and liver strains to clear oxidized fats. The result is familiar, and manifests as sinus congestion, acne, constipation, respiratory stress, and hormonal imbalance. The body becomes a muffled instrument, unable to hear our own intelligence clearly.

Xenogenic Confusion & the Body's Intelligence

Every human cell vibrates with species-specific order. When animal lipopolysaccharides and bovine glycoproteins bind to human receptors, immune surveillance falters. The body interprets our own tissues as infected, perpetuating oxidative stress and chronic fatigue.

Mitochondria, the powerhouses of life, drown in inflammatory debris. Their redox potential declines and ATP production falters. The fatigue many call *"normal aging"* is often this molecular exhaustion. The cost of decoding alien information.

A Conflict of Species

Milk is information transfer. Each sip transmits the cow's biochemical command to *grow, store, and multiply.* Humans requirements are to *differentiate, refine, and evolve.*

To consume another species' milk is to blur that evolutionary boundary and invite code that does not correspond to our genetic library. This is nourishment without alignment and fuel that moves us away from our natural frequency.

The Cost of Borrowed Code

The immune system's vigilance against foreign proteins drains resources from repair and regeneration. The lymph stagnates, liver overworks, and connective tissues lose translucence. Collagen stiffens, eyes dull, and fascia tightens.

What accumulates is not health but heaviness. We experience a slow domestication of human biology by the chemistry of the barnyard.

Returning to Cellular Sovereignty

To abstain from dairy is a form of reclamation that restores ownership of the human bloodstream.

When the xenogenic noise ceases, cellular resonance returns:

• Inflammation subsides.

• Mitochondria rekindle their current.

• Blood regains clarity and charge.

Each molecule once again belongs to the lineage of human evolution, not to the inheritance of herd animals. Health is the body remembering our self.

The True Food of Evolution

If we asked Nature what replaces milk after infancy, she would not answer *"another species' secretion."* She would point to fruit, leaves, seeds, and sunlight. We would be directed to living foods that carry light-encoded energy.

The milks of ascension are coconut water rich in electrolytes, almond oils that lubricate nerve sheaths, chlorophyll that feeds mitochondria, and sap that carries solar information.

We are the only species that drinks the milk of another and the only one that suffers the chronic degenerations that follow, which include cancer, diabetes, atherosclerosis, autoimmune disease, and premature aging.

Milk was intended for the calf, not meant for man. Until humanity remembers that boundary, we will keep paying the price of ignorance in flesh, fatigue, and fog.

Chapter 2: The Truth About Butter, Ghee, & "Sacred" Animal Fats

Why These Fats Do Not Belong in a Healing Body

For a long time, butter and ghee have worn a halo. Raw butter is sold as a *"living superfood."* Ghee is praised as *"sacred"* fuel, and a centerpiece of ancestral wisdom and Ayurvedic tradition. Social media wellness circles exalt these fats as brain food, hormone medicine, and the ultimate *"clean"* calories, but the body responds to molecules, not mythology. When we step away from branding and step inside actual physiology, a different picture emerges.

Butter, ghee, and animal-derived fats, whether raw, grass-fed, or clarified in copper pots, are not neutral, and they are not nourishing in the way people have been told. They are dense, inflammatory, oxidatively fragile fats that overburden the blood, stiffen the arteries, and quietly accelerate aging, especially when heated. This is about chemistry, not dogma.

Raw Butter: The Illusion of "Living" Fat

Raw butter is often defended as a *"whole food,"* full of fat-soluble vitamins, short-chain fatty acids, and beneficial bacteria. What is rarely addressed is what else comes packaged with this product.

The following misalignments are paired with raw butter:

• High saturated fat and cholesterol raise LDL and promote oxidized LDL formation.

• Concentrated hormones and growth factors from lactating animals.

• Persistent environmental toxins (dioxins, PCBs, pesticides, heavy metals) that bioaccumulate in animal fat.

• Endotoxins and microbial fragments that can cross a compromised gut barrier and ignite inflammation.

Even untouched by heat, butter is:

• Devoid of fiber, doing nothing to support microbiome diversity or butyrate production.

• Devoid of antioxidants compared to vibrant plant fats (avocado, olives, nuts, seeds).

• Metabolically acid-forming, increasing the body's need for buffering minerals.

Rawness does not make a harmful profile benign. A raw cigarette is still harmful. A raw chunk of saturated animal fat is still atherosclerotic. *"Enzymes"* and *"life force"* cannot cancel out the hard reality that butter is a dense package of saturated fat and cholesterol in a world already drowning in cardiovascular disease.

Ghee: Clarified Marketing

Ghee is often sold as an upgrade that is *"purer"* than butter because the water and milk solids have been burned off. Ayurvedic language is used to position this product as sattvic, cleansing, and spiritually aligned. Yet the process that creates ghee, which is simmering butter until the water evaporates and milk solids brown, is problematic.

This process creates:

• Oxidized cholesterol (oxysterols).

• Lipid peroxides and aldehydes.

• Advanced lipid oxidation end-products (ALEs).

These compounds:

• Damage cell membranes.

• Disrupt mitochondrial respiration.

• Irritate the endothelium (the inner lining of arteries).

• Contribute to foam cell formation and plaque buildup.

The very browning and nutty aroma people love in ghee is evidence of the Maillard reaction and thermal degradation. This is a perfume of decay dressed up as comfort. Then ghee is often used to fry, sauté, and roast, compounding the problem.

• The higher smoke point is mistaken for safety.

• More contact time at high heat means more oxidation, more aldehydes, more HCAs and PAHs when cooking animal foods.

Ghee is not a neutral ancient remedy. In a modern context of already elevated oxidative stress, this becomes more of an accelerant.

Why "Grass-Fed" Does Not Fix the Biochemistry

Grass-fed butter and ghee may contain slightly higher levels of omega-3s, and certain fat-soluble vitamins compared to grain-fed, but the core issues remain.

These issues include:

• Saturated fat is still saturated fat.

• Dietary cholesterol is still bad cholesterol.

• Oxidized fats are still oxidized fats.

• Environmental contaminants are still stored in animal fat.

Switching to grass-fed is like trading a pack-a-day smoking habit for hand-rolled organic tobacco. The ritual may feel more noble, but the lungs do not care.

What Happens When Animal Fats Are Heated

When butter, ghee, tallow, or lard meet high heat:

1. Fatty acids break down, forming lipid peroxides and highly reactive aldehydes.

2. Cholesterol oxidizes into oxysterols, which embed in cell membranes and disrupt signaling.

3. If used with animal flesh, HCAs (heterocyclic amines) and PAHs (polycyclic aromatic hydrocarbons) form from charred residue.

When these compounds enter the bloodstream, they:

• Increase oxidative stress.

• Impair endothelial function.

• Promote clotting and arterial stiffness.

• Deplete glutathione and other antioxidant reserves.

This is true whether the cooking medium is butter, ghee, or seed oil. The difference is that animal fats start more saturated, cholesterol-heavy, and contaminated, making the damage deeper and more persistent once oxidized. Heated animal fat is not *"real food."* This is molecular wreckage that the liver and arteries are forced to manage.

The Hormonal & Endocrine Fallout

Butter and ghee are not just fat, they are carriers of animal hormones and their metabolites.

These include:

• Estrogenic compounds.

• Progesterone derivatives.

• IGF-1–linked growth signals from dairy.

Chronic intake of these hormone-laden fats:

• Increases estrogen burden and slows clearance through the liver.

• Aggravates hormone-sensitive conditions (fibroids, endometriosis, certain cancers).

• Distorts endocrine signaling in a system already stressed by xenoestrogens and plastics.

Add in the stress hormones (cortisol, adrenaline) that can persist in animal tissues from slaughter, and you have a subtle biochemical cocktail that keeps the nervous system leaning toward fight-or-flight, not rest-and-repair.

The Vascular Reality: Butter & Ghee in the Arteries

Each tablespoon of butter or ghee delivers:

• Saturated fat that stiffens lipid membranes.

• Cholesterol that raises LDL and once oxidized, feeds plaque.

• Thermal byproducts (if cooked) that directly injure the endothelium.

The result over time:

• Decreased nitric oxide, which is the "flow" molecule that keeps arteries relaxed.

• Increased blood viscosity and micro-aggregation of red blood cells.

• Quiet progression of atherosclerosis, often first appearing as erectile dysfunction, cold extremities, sluggish recovery, and subtle cognitive dulling.

While influencers post coffee blended with butter and ghee and call this *"keto clarity,"* the vascular system feels this as slow suffocation.

"But My Ancestors Ate Butter & Ghee"

Your ancestors also:

• Walked more.

• Ate less overall and far fewer processed foods.

• Were not exposed to modern pollution, plastics, microplastics, forever chemicals, synthetic fragrances, and constant stress.

• Had far less access to unlimited calories and constant snacking.

Invoking *"ancestors"* in a completely different toxic landscape is not science. What might have been tolerated in a low-stress, low-toxin, deeply nature-connected life becomes dangerous in a modern, overloaded physiology.

What Actually Nourishes: Living Plant Fats

The body does need fat, but this must be sourced from clean, living, plant-derived fat that comes with protection.

Animal fats (butter, ghee):

• Saturated fat dominant.
• Cholesterol-rich.
• No fiber.
• Sparse antioxidants.
• Often heated → oxidized.
• Hormones and pollutants ride along.

Whole plant fats (as eaten, not refined):

• Avocados, olives, raw nuts, seeds, coconut in moderation.
• Contain fiber, phytosterols, vitamin E, polyphenols.
• Many are eaten raw or gently warmed.
• Support HDL, lower LDL, protect endothelium.
• Feed beneficial microbes when combined with fiber.

These fats:

• Integrate into cell membranes with flexibility, not rigidity.

• Arrive with antioxidant shield molecules that prevent the same oxidative chaos seen with animal fat.

• Do not carry the endocrine confusion of another species.

The Wake-Up Call

We cannot keep pretending that putting melted animal fat into coffee, on vegetables, or into frying pans is some kind of ancestral medicine.

Butter in bulletproof coffee is not biohacking. Ghee in a cast iron pan is not spiritual. Raw butter on sourdough is not regenerative. These are rituals of attachment dressed in the robes of wisdom.

If you want:

• Clear arteries.
• Steady hormones.
• A microbiome that flowers instead of ferments.
• A nervous system that rests instead of fights.
• A heart that beats without sludge in the body rivers.

Then the truth is simple:

Animal fats, whether raw, cooked, clarified, or blessed with a marketing story, do not belong in a healing body.

The body is asking for light, not lard. For chlorophyll, not cholesterol. For living oils wrapped in fiber and antioxidants, not scorched butter sliding down the sides of a pan. When we stop romanticizing animal fat and start listening to blood work, arteries, and lived experience, the madness ends. What remains is the quiet, steady intelligence of a body finally allowed to flow again.

Chapter 3: Casomorphins – The Dairy Drug

The Chemistry of Comfort and the Illusion of Connection

There is a reason people crave cheese more than they crave clarity. Why withdrawal from dairy feels emotional rather than merely dietary. Hidden within the creamy softness of milk is a molecule that speaks to the brain's oldest language. The chemistry of comfort and narcotic whisper of belonging.

Milk was designed to bond a mother and her infant through chemistry. Embedded within this formula is a class of peptides known as β-casomorphins. These are derivatives of the milk protein casein that act directly on the brain's opioid receptors.

In a newborn calf, these molecules induce calmness, stillness, and the deep trust that allows them to nurse and sleep beside their mother. In that sacred design, casomorphins are holy. In the adult human, divorced from the context of infancy and species alignment, these same peptides become chemical captors.

Bondage Biochemistry

When casein is digested, particularly in cheese where casein is condensed nearly ten-fold, β-casomorphin-7 and related peptides are released in the small intestine. These peptides bind to μ-opioid receptors (MORs) in both the gut and the brain. These are the same receptors activated by morphine, heroin, and oxycodone.

This binding induces a mild euphoria, which is experienced as a slowing of respiration and peristalsis, quieting of the mind, and gentle release of dopamine, or the neurotransmitter of reward. The feedback loop is immediate as the consumer is instructed to *eat, soothe, then repeat*. This is why cheese has been called *"dairy crack."*

The potency of cheese is amplified by dehydration and fermentation. As water is removed, casein concentration rises, increasing the dose of casomorphins delivered per bite.

Chronic exposure leads to receptor down-regulation. This is a hallmark of addiction. The body compensates by reducing receptor sensitivity, then requiring larger quantities for the same comfort. When intake stops, withdrawal emerges and this is often paired with irritability, anxiety, and fatigue. The body is not hungry but withdrawing from narcotic nourishment.

Opioids of the Gut and the Mind

The gut-brain axis magnifies this dependency. Roughly ninety percent of the body's serotonin and a dense network of enteric opioid receptors reside in the intestinal wall. Casomorphins act locally before ever reaching the brain, slowing peristalsis and prolonging transit time. The consequence is constipation, fermentation, and the accumulation of toxins that re-enter the bloodstream through enterohepatic recirculation.

The stagnation nurtures endotoxin-producing bacteria (LPS) that leak into circulation, sparking inflammation and emotional dullness. The phrase *"gut feeling"* is literal. When the gut is narcotized, intuition is muffled.

Through the vagus nerve, sedative signals ascend to the brainstem and limbic system, producing the same parasympathetic haze that a narcotic might create. A subtle psychic addiction is then born. One that masquerades as comfort food but functions as a chemical leash.

Emotional Hijacking

Casomorphins shape emotion and hijack the neurochemistry of attachment, binding to the same receptors through which oxytocin and endorphins communicate trust and love. The pleasure of creamy desserts or melted cheese is not emotional healing but neurochemical anesthesia.

These peptides simulate connection while preventing genuine attunement. In doing so, dairy becomes not just a dietary dependency but a substitute for intimacy. A chemical mother whose embrace dulls awareness. This is why quitting dairy often feels like heartbreak. The body grieves the illusion of safety once received from milk's molecular mimicry of affection.

Casomorphins & the Clouding of Consciousness

From a neurological perspective, continual dairy intake maintains a mild, persistent opioid tone. This can be perceived as a constant whisper that dampens cognition. Laboratory studies confirm that β-casomorphin-7 crosses the blood-brain barrier, altering levels of dopamine, serotonin, and acetylcholine.

The effect is subtle but pervasive, and witnessed in slower synaptic firing, reduced focus, and emotional passivity. This biochemical haze is often labeled *"brain fog,"* yet represents a deeper phenomenon. What is truly experienced is the fog of misplaced bonding, and of biochemical comfort replacing conscious vitality.

At the immune level, casomorphins interact with opioid receptors on lymphocytes and macrophages, down-regulating natural killer (NK) cell activity and blunting surveillance against pathogens and tumor cells. The body, lulled into biochemical submission, now forgets alertness. The message of dairy then, is not vitality but is compliance.

The Addiction Cycle

1. Consumption: Milk or cheese enters the body.

2. Conversion: Casein is cleaved into casomorphins.

3. Binding: Opioid receptors in gut and brain are activated.

4. Reward: Dopamine and serotonin deliver transient calm.

5. Tolerance: Receptors desensitize; greater intake required.

6. Withdrawal: Anxiety, lethargy, cravings surface.

7. Relapse: Emotional triggers prompt re-consumption.

This is biochemical conditioning disguised as culture.

Addiction by Design

Processed cheese and dairy desserts are engineered for dependency. Food technologists manipulate fat-to-salt ratios, emulsifiers, and casein concentration to maximize mouthfeel and receptor activation. Every commercial slogan promising *"melty," "creamy,"* or *"indulgent"* is an invocation of neurochemistry, not nourishment.

Even infant formulas derived from cow's milk prime the newborn brain toward casomorphin response, establishing early neuro-associative links between dairy and comfort. The result is a lifetime pattern of self-soothing through incompatible food rather than connection.

The Higher Cost

Excessive casomorphin exposure does more than sedate; this distorts neurotransmitter metabolism. β-Casomorphin-7 inhibits tryptophan transport across the blood-brain barrier, reducing serotonin synthesis and predisposing to depression and anxiety. This also alters the expression of dopamine β-hydroxylase, which is the enzyme converting dopamine to norepinephrine. This results in the flattening of motivation and alertness.

Thus, heavy dairy consumers oscillate between comfort and lethargy, and pleasure and apathy. This is the emotional pendulum of addiction. The price of calm is clarity.

Liberation From the Chemical Comfort

Breaking free from dairy addiction is not an act of punishment but of recalibration. The nervous system must re-sensitize our receptors; the gut must repopulate with living enzymes and flora; and the heart must re-learn real connection. Within weeks of abstinence, opioid receptor density normalizes, bowel motility improves, and dopamine sensitivity resurges. Perception then sharpens, color returns to thought, and we can feel the world again and experience textures of reality once blurred by biochemical sedation.

Freedom from dairy is sovereignty over one's chemistry of bliss and is the difference between peace and paralysis.

From Comfort to Clarity

The child seeks comfort and the awakened being seeks coherence. Casomorphins bind us to the illusion of comfort with a chemical lullaby that soothes but never heals. True nourishment sharpens awareness rather than dulls. To release dairy is to release anesthesia. To return to clarity is to return to consciousness.

Chapter 4: Casein and Cancer

When a Growth Code Becomes a Carcinogenic Signal

Milk is a growth code, not just a beverage. Hidden inside that white liquid is a command written in amino acids to divide, enlarge, multiply, and grow. For an infant calf, this is creation. For an adult human, a seed of degeneration.

The Growth Switch

At the center of dairy's danger is casein, the dominant protein in cow's milk. Casein makes up roughly eighty percent of milk's total protein load and serves one primary purpose, which is to accelerate cellular growth. This happens by activating the body's IGF-1 (Insulin-Like Growth Factor-1) and mTOR (mechanistic Target of Rapamycin) pathways. These are two of the most powerful anabolic signaling systems known to biology.

• **IGF-1** tells cells to divide and to resist apoptosis, the natural self-destruct mechanism that prevents cancer.

• **mTORC1** is the throttle on protein synthesis and cell replication. When locked "on," our body loses the rhythm of renewal and rest (suppressed autophagy and heightened cell-cycle drive).

Every glass of milk is an instruction to grow, not selectively or intelligently, but indiscriminately. An additional mechanism is that casein supplies abundant branched-chain amino acids (BCAAs) and leucine, potent activators of mTORC1 via Rag GTPases and S6K1. In parallel, dairy increases circulating IGF-1, which signals through PI3K→Akt→mTORC1, inhibits FoxO tumor-suppressive transcription factors, and reduces autophagy, together creating a biochemical soil where initiated cells expand rather than self-correct.

From Nourishment to Neoplasia

In a human adult whose developmental growth is long complete, this constant stimulation has consequences. IGF-1 levels rise in the bloodstream after dairy intake, and with them rises the risk of breast, prostate, ovarian, and colorectal cancers. Laboratory and animal studies reveal that casein acts as a tumor promoter, not by introducing carcinogens, but by accelerating the proliferation of mutated cells that already exist.

In *The China Study*, Dr. T. Colin Campbell demonstrated that rats fed casein-rich diets experienced rapid tumor growth when exposed to aflatoxin B1. When casein was removed, tumors regressed. Casein was not the match that lit the fire but was the oxygen that kept the flame burning.

Prospective cohorts repeatedly link higher IGF-1, and dairy intake, to increased risk of prostate, breast, and colorectal cancers. While confounding exists, the consistency of the IGF-axis association and the strength of the mTORC1 rationale provide a biologically credible bridge from diet to disease.

Hormonal Hijacking

Dairy carries a distinct hormonal payload. Even milk from cows never treated with rBGH contains estrogens, progesterone, cortisol, and growth factors produced during pregnancy. These hormones are biologically active in humans. Steroid hormones survive pasteurization and digestion largely intact as estrone sulfate and other conjugates that are readily absorbed.

They are then able to bind to receptor sites in breast, prostate, uterine, and ovarian tissue, amplifying cell-division signals already ignited by casein/IGF-1.

• In men, this infiltration lowers androgenic tone and stresses the prostate microenvironment.

• In women, this exaggerates estrogen dominance, manifesting as fibroids, cysts, endometriosis, and a higher hormonal proliferative drive.

The body becomes a field of overstimulated cells waiting for instruction to mutate.

Acid and Oxidation: The Soil of Disease

Casein digestion leaves behind acidic metabolites, uric acid, sulfuric acid, and lactic residues that the body must neutralize using alkaline mineral reserves. Calcium is drawn from bones and teeth while magnesium is depleted from tissues. This mineral robbery creates a terrain where oxygen delivery falters, red blood cells aggregate, and anaerobic metabolism, the hallmark of malignant tissue, takes hold.

As Otto Warburg described nearly a century ago, cancer cells thrive where oxygen is scarce and acidity prevails. Dairy, rich in casein and saturated fat, cultivates precisely that terrain by increasing acid load and lipid peroxidation, while suppressing autophagic cleanup.

Pasteurization and Protein Corruption

When milk is heated during pasteurization (HTST, UHT), the proteins denature and cross-link, forming advanced glycation end-products (AGEs) and advanced lipoxidation end-products (ALEs) that generate reactive oxygen species (ROS) and ignite inflammatory cascades.

Denatured casein becomes more immunogenic, provoking antibody formation and chronic immune activation, both conditions that deplete the body's surveillance capacity against malignant cells and impair immunoediting (elimination→ equilibrium→ escape).

What began as nourishment now behaves as a slow toxin, eroding redox equilibrium and tilting tissues toward proliferation without repair.

Calcium's Deception

Industry propaganda insists that dairy *"builds strong bones,"* yet epidemiological data reveal the opposite, indicating that the highest dairy-consuming nations often experience the greatest incidence of osteoporosis and hip fracture. The acidic aftermath of casein metabolism dissolves bone matrix faster than dairy calcium can replace.

This calcium loss not only weakens structure but also deposits calcified debris in soft tissues, arteries, joints, and kidneys, where this fuels inflammation and stiffness, compounding the oxidative stress that feeds malignant change. Ectopic calcification is a pro-inflammatory, pro-tumor microenvironment.

The Casein–IGF Axis and Metabolic Cancer

Chronic stimulation of the IGF-1 receptor does not merely encourage cell growth but suppresses autophagy. This is the self-cleansing process that removes damaged mitochondria and misfolded proteins. Without autophagy, mutations accumulate, mitochondrial efficiency declines, and genomic instability increases.

This same mTORC1/IGF-1 pathway underlies insulin resistance and Type 2 diabetes, both recognized as pre-cancerous metabolic states. High insulin and IGF-1 synergize to accelerate PI3K→Akt signaling, inhibit AMPK, and reduce p53/FoxO activity, each being key brakes on carcinogenesis. In this way, dairy's growth signals weave through the modern epidemics of obesity, diabetes, hormonal disease, and cancer and share one biochemical thread, the unrelenting presence of IGF-1 activation.

Immune Surveillance, Inflammation, & Tumor Niche

Beyond proliferation, casein-driven endotoxemia (via high-fat dairy meals) elevates LPS, engaging TLR4 and boosting IL-6 and TNF-α. These cytokines support tumor survival, angiogenesis, and immune evasion. Concurrently, opioid peptides from dairy (β-casomorphins) down-regulate NK-cell activity, dulling the innate immune response that recognizes transformed cells. The tumor is not only growing but is also becoming less visible to the body's sentinels.

A Sacred Misalignment

In nature, growth and decay are balanced. Creation yields to rest and expansion yields to refinement. Casein abolishes that rhythm, keeping the biological accelerator pressed down long after the journey should have slowed.

To feed the human body cow's milk is to feed the chemistry of growth without wisdom. The calf requires bulk, while the human requires balance. When the chemistry of bulk is imposed on the organism of consciousness, the result is proliferation without purpose and tumors of flesh mirroring the tumors of a culture addicted to excess.

The Healing Countercurrent

When dairy leaves the diet, the body begins a quiet revolution.

• IGF-1 levels fall within days to weeks.

• mTORC1 activity normalizes; AMPK rises.

• Autophagy resumes, sweeping away damaged cells.

• Systemic acid load declines, oxygen tension rises, and immune clarity returns.

• Cravings fade, energy stabilizes, and eyes brighten with the voltage of unburdened biology.

In Summary

Casein is not a nutrient but a signal. In infancy that signal means life. In adulthood this becomes an echo of growth that no longer serves evolution.

To silence this is to reclaim the equilibrium of the human temple, fostering a chemistry aligned with consciousness rather than consumption.

Chapter 5: The Mucus Matrix

Within the cathedral of the human body, rivers of light and lymph flow through every corridor that are washing, cleansing, and renewing the architecture of life. When those rivers are pure, energy sings. When they thicken, stagnation begins.

Dairy is the great coagulator that turns the crystalline currents of human physiology into sludge, veiling vitality beneath layers of mucus and fatigue. What appears on the surface as sinus congestion or skin eruption is merely the body's weeping, or the overflow of an internal swamp.

The Body's Rivers

The lymphatic system is the unsung circulatory network that filters metabolic debris, neutralizes pathogens, and transports immune cells. Lymph moves through pressure, breath, and muscle contraction as a fluid symphony dependent on rhythm and clarity.

Dairy disrupts that rhythm. The dense fats and glue-like proteins, particularly casein, generate mucoproteins when digested. These mucoproteins thicken the lymph, much like cream poured into clear water. The lymphatic system then becomes sluggish, and the immune system must divert energy to manage this viscous tide.

The result is swollen lymph nodes, fatigue, sluggish bowels, recurring colds, and a film that lingers in the throat after milk or cheese. This is the body's first sign of suffocation.

The Chemistry of Congestion

When casein reaches the stomach, the protein encounters hydrochloric acid and enzymes like pepsin, forming a dense curd. This coagulum digests slowly, releasing amines such as *histamine, cadaverine,* and *putrescine* through bacterial fermentation. These compounds irritate mucous membranes, causing histamine release, swelling, and fluid secretion. The body reacts as though under attack. The sinuses flood, the bronchi narrow, and the gut inflames.

Meanwhile, dairy fats suppress bile flow, limiting fat emulsification and further clogging elimination pathways. The stagnation of bile leads to the stagnation of everything, including toxins reabsorbed, hormones recirculated, and lymph thickened.

This internal congestion manifests as external heaviness and is expressed through bloating, puffiness, eczema, chronic sinusitis, and that dull, congested tone in the skin.

The Protective Fog

Mucus is the body's defense and is not to be mistaken as the villain. When cells are assaulted by irritants, the mucosal lining from the nasal cavity to the colon secretes a glycoprotein gel called mucin to trap and escort out foreign matter. When dairy consumption is chronic, the secretion never stops and the protection becomes pathology.

This sticky matrix traps bacteria, endotoxins, and undigested proteins, creating an internal compost heap that perpetuates inflammation. In the intestines, this biofilm fosters anaerobic bacterial overgrowth, reducing oxygen and impairing nutrient absorption. The result is a bloodstream starved of minerals yet flooded with metabolic waste.

Respiratory Repercussions

In the respiratory tract, the pattern repeats. The inhaled world meets the dairy-loaded bloodstream, and the lungs become the arena for excretion. The body tries to eliminate mucoproteins through bronchial and sinus discharge, which explains the chronic phlegm and *"post-nasal drip"* often dismissed as seasonal allergies.

At the cellular level, these secretions reduce alveolar surface area, limiting oxygen exchange. Chronic hypoxia follows where there is a subtle lack of oxygen that the body compensates for by increasing heart rate and stress hormones. Over time, this low-oxygen state dulls cognition, mood, and mitochondrial output. This is not just a stuffy nose but is biochemical suffocation.

Lymphatic Burden & the Brain Fog Connection

Recent research confirms that the glymphatic system, known as the brain's lymphatic network, clears waste from neural tissues during deep sleep. When systemic lymph is congested, cerebral detox slows, leading to neuroinflammation and the heavy fog so many experience after consuming dairy.

The inflammatory molecules *IL-6* and *TNF-α* rise in response to casein fragments and bacterial endotoxins, crossing the blood-brain barrier and impairing synaptic signaling. This is more of a neuromolecular haze than fog.

In Ayurvedic and Taoist terms, this is *ama,* or stagnation of subtle fluids. In modern biochemistry, this is finally recognized as impaired drainage, oxidative stress, and toxic biofilm accumulation.

The Lymph–Liver Loop

The liver filters what the lymph delivers. When the lymph is thick with dairy residues, bile becomes viscous and overloaded. Biliary congestion follows, impairing fat metabolism and detoxification. The feedback loop intensifies as the body recycles waste hormones like estrogen and cortisol, amplifying fatigue, anxiety, and inflammation.

This is why quitting dairy often triggers short-lived "detox symptoms," often expressed through the release of stored mucus and reactivation of lymphatic flow. The body is not sick but is *remembering how to cleanse.*

The Path Back to Clarity

Elimination is liberation. When dairy is removed, lymphatic rhythm returns. Within days, sinuses clear. Within weeks, breath deepens. Within months, the skin glows. The taste buds then sharpen to subtler sweetness and the hidden symphony of plants.

Supportive allies include:

• **Raw vegetable juices** (celery, cucumber, parsley): natural diuretics for lymph flow.

• **Ginger, turmeric, and cayenne**: bio-catalysts for microcirculation.

• **Enzyme-rich foods** (pineapple, papaya, sprouts): dissolve residual mucoproteins.

• **Movement, deep breathing, and sweating**: the trinity of drainage.

When the body's rivers flow freely, the spirit's current follows. What begins as physical detox becomes emotional clarity and a release of the density that dulls perception.

Reflection

On a planetary scale, the mucus matrix mirrors humanity's ecological congestion. Rivers are choked with waste, skies are heavy with particulates, and oceans slick with oil. As within, so without. When we free our inner waters, we participate in the Earth's own purification.

Chapter 6: Homogenization, Pasteurization & Bacterial Decay

In the field of modern dairy, the white liquid of the cow is not simply collected but is processed, engineered, compressed, and twisted. The raw milk of nature passes through machines, heat, pressure, and chemical horizons. What emerges is not the fluid of the cow, but a *manufactured signal* masquerading as nourishment.

This chapter lifts the lid on the three processing pillars that include homogenization, pasteurization, and the insidious breeding ground of latent bacterial decay. Each is a transformation of milk's chemistry, and each carries consequences for the body's chemistry in turn.

Homogenization: The Fat Globule Revolution

Homogenization is the mechanical splitting of milk's fat globules into minute particles, forced through tiny apertures under high pressure so that the cream no longer rises and the fluid remains *"homogeneous."*

Under this pressure, the native milk-fat globule membrane (MFGM) is ruptured. The fat droplets swell in surface area, proteins (especially casein) re-interface at the droplet surface, and the physical architecture of milk is fundamentally changed. Proponents of milk's nutritional quality argue this only affects texture and shelf life; critics say the new structure invites pathologic integration into human physiology.

One often-cited hypothesis (though still contested) is that the enzyme Xanthine Oxidase (XO), originally present in the fat globule membranes, becomes encapsulated in liposomes during homogenization and may be absorbed intact, entering the human circulation and oxidizing lipids, depleting plasmalogens in arterial walls, and contributing to atherosclerosis.

However, the scientific consensus is far from settled. Reviews state that *"absorption of dietary xanthine oxidase has not been demonstrated"* and that *"neither liposome formation, nor absorption, has been demonstrated."* Yet, even if that specific mechanism remains speculative, the broader change in molecular architecture demands attention.

The fat globules now exist in a form the body did not evolve to process. They are smaller, more abundant, and more protein-bound. They may pass the gut, engage the lymphatics, and burden the body's clearance systems differently. In short, homogenization creates a milk that is physically different from nature's design.

Pasteurization: Heat, Denature, Disempower

Pasteurization is the thermal assault on milk, where the fluid is typically heated to ~72 °C for fifteen seconds (HTST) or other time-temperature combinations. The stated goal is to kill pathogens, yet in the process, the milk's living enzymes, subtle lipid membranes, and delicate proteins are irreversibly altered. Studies show that the activity of xanthine oxidase (XO) in milk decreases with increasing heat. Only high-temperature short time (HTST) preserves significant activity, while ultra-high temperature (UHT) essentially eliminates. In other words, heat does not just sterilize but reconfigures.

The downstream effects of this molecular disruption include:

• **Protein denaturation**: Casein micelles lose their natural configuration, exposing hydrophobic segments, promoting aggregation, and potentially increasing immunogenicity.

• **Loss of beneficial enzymes**: Enzymes such as lactoperoxidase, phosphatase, and vitamin-carriers are destroyed, removing the 'living' quality of milk.

• **Lipid oxidation**: Heat accelerates oxidation of the fat globules, forming lipid peroxides and advanced glycation end-products (AGEs) that invade cell membranes and provoke inflammatory responses.

When you drink pasteurized milk, you are not drinking the fluid of the cow, you are drinking the *remains* of the cow's milk after mechanical and thermal violence. This has implications at the cell-level that include oxidized lipids, damaged proteins, and compromised clearance.

Bacterial Decay & Endotoxin Load: The Hidden Burden

Even beyond the processing lies a biological tension of bacteria, endotoxins, and microbial fragments. Whether raw or processed, dairy remains a substrate, and the body must handle the microbial by-products.

• Raw milk is subject to contamination by pathogens (U.S. Food & Drug Administration warns of multiple outbreaks). U.S. Food and Drug Administration.

• Processed milk, despite sterilization efforts, still carries lipopolysaccharides (LPS), bacterial fragments, micro-vesicles and oxidized proteins that enter the gut, activate Toll-like receptors (TLRs), provoke systemic inflammation, and burden the liver-lymph axis.

These endotoxins and fragments increase gut permeability ("leaky gut"), trigger immune activation, and throttle mitochondrial efficiency. The result is fatigue, systemic inflammation, mood disorders, and the cellular wear-and-tear that accelerates aging.

Processing may reduce the microbial load but cannot restore the fluid to original alive-state. Instead, this leaves a chemical skeleton, prepared to provoke rather than nourish.

Chyle, Lymph & the Sacred Flow Interrupted

Chyle is the milky fluid produced by the gut during digestion of fats that is meant to carry nutrient-lipids, immune markers, and growth factors into the body's lymphatic network. Processed milk alters the quality of this chyle. The fats are oxidized, proteins are denatured, and enzymatic complement is lost. Therefore, lymph must carry burden instead of blessing.

When the lymph becomes heavy, the body's filtration systems (lymph nodes, spleen, and liver) become overloaded. Clearance slows, residues remain, and the long-term effect is the same as the slow drift into cellular stagnation. This leads to accumulation of denatured proteins, oxidized lipids, immune 'fog', and age acceleration.

When the body is designed to run like a river, processed dairy forces internal fluid to slog like a swamp.

The Myth of "Raw" or "Grass-Fed" Milk

The dairy world often counters critiques with *"raw milk"* or *"grass-fed milk"* as superior, but the chemistry remains in fat globules, casein proteins, lactose, and growth factors from another species. The processing may be lighter, but the biology remains foreign.

"Raw" milk still carries foreign bacteria, fosters acid-forming residues, and introduces xenogenic growth factors. The notion of a 'pure' milk is misleading because what matters is *species-specificity*, not marketing veneer.

Thus, whether homogenized & pasteurized, or labelled "raw/grass-fed," the issue remains where our physiology is being asked to integrate fluids designed for bovines.

The Return Path: Reclaiming the Stream

Reversal begins when one stops consuming these processed dairy forms and instead supports the body's natural fluid dynamics.

• **Antioxidant & enzyme-rich foods**: sprouts, chlorophyll-rich greens, fresh juices to counter oxidized lipids.

• **Movement & lymphatic activation**: rebounding, dry-brushing, sauna to support lymph clearance.

• **Gut-repair protocol**: fermented plant foods, elimination of LPS triggers, rebuilding tight-junction integrity.

• **Rich, unprocessed fats from plants**: avocado, coconut, olive; these fatty acids integrate cleanly, without the mechanical/thermal trauma of processed dairy.

The body remembers flow. Once the external assault (processed milk) is removed, the internal rivers begin to cleanse themselves. Cells begin to shed the sediment. Tissues regain their transparency.

Summary & Reflection

In the chemistry of the modern dairy industry, we witness three key interventions: mechanical stress (homogenization), thermal stress (pasteurization), and microbial residue (endotoxin load). Each distorts the original design of milk, which is a fluid intended to nourish within species, into a fluid that burdens across species.

When we drink processed cow's milk, we ingest not only the cow's growth fluid but also the products of mechanical force, heat damage, and microbial fragment. The rivers of the body are meant to flow; processed dairy makes them stagnate. To reclaim vitality, we must step out of the engineered white lie and return to true fluids of life.

Chapter 7: Acid, Endotoxins & Inflammation

The human body is a symphony of balance. Every cell, enzyme, and organ performs a song within the narrowest range of pH. This is an orchestra tuned to 7.4. When that balance falters, vitality fades.

Dairy, despite the creamy softness, strikes a dissonant note in this harmony. This is not alkaline, as the appearance might suggest, but acid-forming. Think of this as a biochemical thief that robs the bones to buffer the residue, leaving behind the ashes of inflammation, soot of oxidation, and silent noise of disease.

The Acid-Ash Aftermath

When animal proteins like casein are metabolized, they release sulfuric, phosphoric, and uric acids. These are each acidic end-products that must be neutralized to maintain blood pH. To do so, the body extracts calcium, magnesium, and potassium from bones and tissues. The result is temporary stability but long-term depletion.

This process, known as the acid-ash hypothesis, is supported by decades of biochemical research showing that diets high in animal protein correlate with increased urinary calcium excretion and bone demineralization.

Contrary to the marketing myth, milk leaches from and weakens bones, while not contributing in any way to the building processes. Calcium that enters through the mouth exits through the urine, escorted by the acids you neutralize.

The loss is not only skeletal but also cellular. Chronic acidosis impairs mitochondrial efficiency, reduces ATP generation, and promotes the conversion of healthy aerobic respiration into anaerobic fermentation. This is the same metabolic shift Dr. Otto Warburg identified as the foundation of cancer.

Endotoxins: The Invisible Poison

Inside every sip of milk, raw or pasteurized, is a microscopic battlefield. When bacteria die (whether from heat, age, or digestion), they release lipopolysaccharides (LPS), these are fragments of their cell walls known collectively as endotoxins.

These endotoxins are not destroyed by pasteurization. The heat merely disarms the living cell but leaves a toxic skeleton intact. Once ingested, LPS travels through the digestive tract, sometimes breaching the intestinal barrier and entering circulation. There, they bind to Toll-Like Receptor 4 (TLR4) on immune cells, igniting a systemic inflammatory cascade.

The result is elevated levels of C-reactive protein (CRP), interleukin-6 (IL-6), and tumor necrosis factor-alpha (TNF-α). These are cytokines that drive fatigue, insulin resistance, depression, and chronic disease. This inflammation is experienced as exhaustion, stiffness, and brain fog.

Leaky Gut, Leaky Mind

The intestinal lining is a single-cell membrane. The film is thin enough to tear at a whisper. When dairy-derived endotoxins and casein fragments encounter this lining, the immune system launches antibodies that mistake the body's own cells for invaders. Tight junctions between intestinal cells loosen, allowing molecules to slip through into the bloodstream. This is intestinal permeability, or *"leaky gut."*

Once the gates open, the blood becomes polluted with what the gut was meant to keep out. Immune cells misfire and inflammation spreads to joints, skin, and even the brain. The gut, once a guardian, becomes a sieve.

In this state, dairy's proteins and bacterial fragments act like spies, crossing borders and whispering confusion into the immune code. Over time, the miscommunication becomes chronic, evolving into autoimmune disorders such as rheumatoid arthritis, lupus, multiple sclerosis, and inflammatory bowel disease.

The Depression Connection

Inflammation goes beyond the physical body and crosses into consciousness. Elevated endotoxin load suppresses serotonin production, disrupts tryptophan metabolism, and triggers kynurenine pathway activation, creating a biochemical detour that generates neurotoxic metabolites.

The same LPS molecules that inflame the gut also inflame the brain. When microglial cells, which are the brain's immune sentinels, detect LPS, they release reactive oxygen species (ROS) that damage neurons and blunt neurotransmission. The result is irritability, the fog of fatigue, and hopelessness often misdiagnosed as depression.

Dairy, being rich in arachidonic acid and inflammatory triggers, fuels this cascade. Each bite of cheese or spoonful of yogurt feeds the chemistry of low mood.

IGF-1, mTOR, and the Inflammatory Growth Loop

Inflammation is destructive and proliferative. Casein and dairy hormones elevate IGF-1 (Insulin-Like Growth Factor 1), which activates the mTOR pathway. This is a master regulator of growth and metabolism. Chronic mTOR activation drives cellular proliferation and inhibits autophagy, the body's mechanism for recycling damaged cells. Without autophagy, inflammation festers and the body cannot clean up.

The result is premature aging, cancerous potential, and metabolic stagnation. We foster the conditions for a body stuck in perpetual growth without refinement.

Nature's intelligence designed growth for infancy, not for eternity. When dairy keeps mTOR locked *"on,"* the body forgets how to rest, renew, and release.

The Microbial Mirror

The bacteria within us mirror the terrain we cultivate. A plant-rich, fiber-fed microbiome produces short-chain fatty acids (SCFAs) like butyrate. These are anti-inflammatory compounds that feed colon cells and stabilize the gut barrier. A dairy-fed microbiome, however, shifts toward acid-forming bacteria that thrive on putrefaction such as *Clostridium, Escherichia,* and *Proteus.*

These microbes generate ammonia, amines, and hydrogen sulfide. Each are toxic gases that burden the liver and dull the brain. The gut becomes a swamp instead of a garden.

The Spiritual Biology of Inflammation

Inflammation is the body's cry for clarity and can be viewed as sacred fire meant to purify that is now trapped in a cycle of irritation. When the lymph thickens, breath shortens, and blood loses sparkle, the soul begins to suffocate within our vessel.

To cleanse the body of dairy is to let that sacred fire burn clean again. The acid clears, lymph flows, and inner waters remember light.

Recovery: Neutralizing the Fire

• **Plant alkalinity**: Green juices, mineral broths, and fruits replenish potassium and magnesium, restoring cellular pH.

• **Antioxidants**: Vitamins C and E, polyphenols from berries, neutralize ROS and stabilize mitochondria.

• **Gut restoration**: L-glutamine, slippery elm, and prebiotic fibers rebuild intestinal integrity.

• **Oxygenation**: Deep breathing, sauna, and ozone therapy renew aerobic metabolism.

• **Purification therapies**: Colon hydrotherapy, herbal binders, and clean hydration assist in clearing endotoxin burden.

Inflammation cannot coexist with flow. When the fluids move, the fire cools, and the body reclaims rhythm.

In Summary

The story of dairy is the story of imbalance. There is acid where there should be neutrality, inflammation where there should be regeneration, and growth where there should be rest.

Endotoxins and acidosis are not isolated effects. These are signals of dissonance between species, chemistry, and consciousness. To heal, we must realign with our design and learn to feed the blood with light, not residue.

Chapter 8: Fat Cells, Insulin & Intramyocellular Lipids

The modern epidemic of fatigue, obesity, and diabetes is not born of sugar alone, but is primarily born of a *sludge* that consists of fats and proteins that never belonged to the human bloodstream. At the molecular level, dairy is not a source of energy but of interference.

Dairy fats lodge within cells, the proteins block gates of metabolism, and hormones confuse the language of insulin. The result is a global condition of cellular suffocation lurking within bodies full of calories but starved for current.

The Hidden Burden of Milk Fat

Cow's milk fat is heavy in saturated fatty acids, particularly palmitic acid (C16:0), myristic acid (C14:0), and stearic acid (C18:0). These fats differ markedly from the unsaturated, oxygen-friendly lipids found in fruits, seeds, and nuts. When absorbed, they enter the bloodstream in chylomicrons and are stored in adipocytes. These are the fat cells that line our body's connective tissue.

Each adipocyte is an endocrine organ in miniature, secreting hormones such as leptin, adiponectin, and resistin that regulate appetite and insulin sensitivity. Dairy fat distorts this hormonal orchestra, as palmitic acid suppresses adiponectin (which promotes insulin sensitivity) and increases resistin (which induces resistance).

Thus, every serving of butter or cream tightens the body's metabolic circuits, thereby blocking the conversation between insulin and its receptor.

Intramyocellular Lipids: Fat Inside the Muscle

Healthy muscle tissue burns glucose efficiently, but when saturated fats from dairy accumulate within muscle fibers, they form droplets known as intramyocellular lipids (IMCLs). These are considered by many real health experts as a leading cause of diabetes. The droplets interfere with insulin-signaling cascades by activating protein kinase C (PKC) and serine phosphorylation of the insulin receptor substrate (IRS-1).

In practical terms, insulin knocks on the cell's door, but the signal is jammed. Glucose cannot enter. The pancreas compensates by releasing more insulin, creating hyperinsulinemia, which drives hunger, fat storage, and eventual burnout of the β-cells. This process, which is invisible and slow, is the metabolic shadow of dairy and the creation of insulin resistance inside living tissue.

The IGF-1 Parallel

As described in earlier chapters, dairy's natural growth factor IGF-1 amplifies this process by mimicking insulin. The two molecules share structural homology, and IGF-1 can bind to insulin receptors, producing erratic glucose uptake. Meanwhile, elevated IGF-1 levels block lipolysis (fat breakdown) and promote lipogenesis (fat creation).

The outcome is paradoxical. More fat is stored and less energy is liberated. The body becomes an engine idling in thick oil with plenty of fuel, but no ignition.

The Arachidonic Acid Angle

Beyond the saturated fats, dairy carries arachidonic acid, an omega-6 fatty acid that serves as the raw material for inflammatory prostaglandins (PGE_2) and leukotrienes. These mediators heighten pain sensitivity, vascular inflammation, and depressive tendencies. In metabolic tissues, they reduce insulin sensitivity by impairing receptor function and altering membrane fluidity. In essence, dairy fat *sabotages* the very receptor that governs energy balance.

Mitochondria in Muck

Inside the cell, mitochondria are designed to burn clean fuels like glucose and unsaturated fats. When saturated dairy fats dominate, β-oxidation becomes incomplete, producing ceramides and diacylglycerols (DAGs). These are lipotoxic intermediates that poison mitochondrial membranes. Ceramides are now recognized as major drivers of insulin resistance, as research shows they block Akt phosphorylation, which is a key step in glucose transport.

Thus, dairy's biochemistry literally dims the cell's fire, impairing oxygen flow, reducing ATP, and fostering fatigue. The human engine begins to sputter.

From Cream to Crisis

Epidemiological studies link high dairy intake with increased risk of Type 2 diabetes, cardiovascular disease, and obesity. While some industry-funded trials argue otherwise, they often isolate calcium or whey peptides and ignore the holistic chemistry of real-world dairy. The full cocktail of fats, growth hormones, and acid residues that accompany every glass of milk are virtually ignored.

The truth, observed across independent analyses, is that dairy consumption correlates with insulin resistance, higher fasting insulin, and elevated inflammatory markers.

The Endocrine Hijack

As adipose tissue expands under dairy's influence, more leptin is secreted, but paradoxically, the brain becomes leptin-resistant. The appetite-control centers in the hypothalamus no longer respond, perpetuating hunger.

Meanwhile, estrogenic compounds in dairy fat derived from pregnant cows further confuse metabolic regulation, especially in women. The hormonal misalignment mirrors the biochemical one when people are overfed, undernourished, and hormonally disoriented.

Purification & Reversal

The human body, miraculous in memory, can recover from this metabolic murk. When dairy is removed and replaced with plant-based lipids, insulin sensitivity begins to rebound within weeks.

• **Omega-3s** from flax and chia restore membrane fluidity.

• **Polyphenols** from berries and green tea quench inflammatory prostaglandins.

• **Fiber-rich foods** improve gut microbiota composition, lowering circulating LPS and restoring leptin sensitivity.

• **Movement and sweating** oxidize intramyocellular fats, clearing the muscle of its metabolic ghosts.

As fat within cells drains, our spark returns. The body remembers how to listen again as insulin's whisper is heard.

Reflection

Milk fat was designed to build a calf, not to sustain human consciousness. When that foreign fuel infiltrates the human body, every metabolic command gets confused. The consequence is visible not only on the scale but in the eyes, on the skin, and in the spirit. To abandon dairy is to invite light back into the cell.

Chapter 9: The Arachidonic Acid Link

How Dairy Fuels Depression, Inflammation & the Chemistry of Suffering

There are fires that heal and fires that harm. Some warmth clears infection, sparks immunity, and restores rhythm. The fire born of dairy is a slow smolder that never dies, living quietly in the membranes of our cells. This flame has a name, arachidonic acid. This is the fat of fury and the biochemical signal of pain, anxiety, and unrest.

Arachidonic Acid: The Fire Within

Every cell in the human body is wrapped in a delicate phospholipid membrane. This serves as a living border that decides what comes in and what leaves. Within those phospholipids lie stored fatty acids that are basically reservoirs of potential energy and chemical communication. One of these, arachidonic acid (AA), is a 20-carbon omega-6 polyunsaturated fat.

Under stress, whether physical, emotional, or dietary, the enzyme phospholipase A_2 cleaves AA from the membrane, sending this acid into the cytoplasm. Once freed, AA becomes the raw material for eicosanoids. These are signaling molecules that regulate inflammation, blood flow, and immunity.

These eicosanoids, which include prostaglandins, thromboxanes, and leukotrienes, are not inherently evil. In acute injury, they initiate healing. When the tissue pool of arachidonic acid is excessive, every stressor from each meal, anxious thought, or surge of cortisol releases more than the body can use. The result is chronic activation so extreme that inflammation becomes a lifestyle and pain is implemented as a personality.

How Dairy Amplifies the Arachidonic Pool

Cow's milk fat, butter, cheese, and cream contain both arachidonic acid and the precursor linoleic acid (18:2 n-6). Humans convert linoleic acid to AA via the enzyme $\Delta 5$-desaturase, an activity enhanced by insulin and saturated fat, which are both elevated after dairy consumption.

A single ounce of cheese or a tablespoon of butter may seem harmless, but over weeks these sources saturate red-blood-cell membranes with AA. Studies confirm that habitual consumers of dairy exhibit a higher AA: EPA ratio. This is a predictive marker of systemic inflammation.

This imbalance tips the eicosanoid orchestra toward pro-inflammatory prostaglandin E_2 (PGE_2) and leukotriene B_4 (LTB_4), both molecules that whisper pain into joints, confusion into neurons, and exhaustion into mitochondria.

The Inflammatory Cascade

Once released from the membrane, AA follows two main enzymatic fates:

1. The Cyclooxygenase (COX) Pathway $\rightarrow$ Produces prostaglandins and thromboxanes.

- *PGE_2*: Triggers fever, pain, and vascular dilation.
- *TXA_2*: Stimulates platelet aggregation and vasoconstriction.

2. The Lipoxygenase (LOX) Pathway $\rightarrow$ Produces leukotrienes and hydroxyeicosatetraenoic acids (HETEs).

- *LTB_4*: Attracts immune cells, perpetuating inflammation.
- *5-HETE*: Induces oxidative stress and tissue damage.

When these molecules flood the bloodstream daily, as they do in heavy dairy eaters, inflammation becomes permanent and the immune system is corroded.

From Gut to Mind: The Inflammation of Emotion

Inflammation travels through the blood and into the brain. Arachidonic acid–derived eicosanoids cross the blood-brain barrier, activating microglial cells that are the immune sentinels of the nervous system. These microglia release reactive oxygen species (ROS) and nitric oxide, which impair synaptic transmission and lower the firing of serotonin neurons.

Simultaneously, inflammatory cytokines such as IL-1β, IL-6, and TNF-α upregulate the enzyme indoleamine-2,3-dioxygenase (IDO), diverting tryptophan, the amino acid precursor of serotonin, into the kynurenine pathway. The by-product, quinolinic acid, is a neurotoxin that overstimulates NMDA receptors and leads to depressive, anxious, and irritable states.

Thus, the chemistry of dairy becomes the chemistry of despair. Mood darkens from the storm raging at the molecular level.

The Pain Connection

The same prostaglandins that distort mood also sensitize nociceptors, the pain-sensing neurons. PGE_2 lowers their firing threshold so that mild pressure or temperature feels like pain. People living with chronic headaches, fibromyalgia, menstrual cramps, and arthritis often describe a kind of *"dull ache that never leaves."*

Dairy intensifies this ache by feeding the biochemical machinery that is the hidden hand behind countless bottles of ibuprofen.

Endothelial Dysfunction & the Silent Heart

In arteries, AA-derived thromboxane A_2 tightens blood vessels and promotes clot formation. At the same time, oxidized dairy fats impair endothelial nitric oxide synthase (eNOS), reducing nitric-oxide production. Nitric oxide is important because this is the molecule that keeps vessels flexible and blood pressure steady.

Over time, this dual assault breeds endothelial dysfunction, and this is the root of hypertension and atherosclerosis. The vessel wall becomes brittle as the once-silken interior turns rough, inviting cholesterol and calcium to cling. The dairy consumer may never see this happening but will experience fatigue, cold hands, or loss of stamina.

Hormonal Hijack of the Reproductive System

Prostaglandins derived from arachidonic acid also govern uterine contractions. Excess PGE_2 is linked to dysmenorrhea (painful menstruation) and endometriosis. In both men and women, inflammatory prostaglandins interfere with steroid hormone synthesis, reducing fertility and libido.

Whether raw or pasteurized, dairy carries bovine estrogens and progesterone that further amplify this imbalance, creating hormonal cross-talk that confuses the body's natural cycles. Inflammation and endocrine disruption become twin flames. One chemical and the other is hormonal.

Arachidonic Acid & the Mitochondrial Spiral

Inflammatory cytokines generated by excess AA disrupt mitochondrial membranes. When ROS outpace antioxidant defenses, the inner membrane's cardiolipin, which is rich in unsaturated fatty acids, becomes oxidized, impairing electron transport. ATP then drops, and the cell shifts toward anaerobic metabolism. This explains the paradox of modern fatigue where there is abundant calories, but no current. Dairy fills the body with fuel that short-circuits its own energy production.

Breaking the Cycle: Restoring the Ratio

The key to ending inflammation is not merely removing AA but restoring balance. The opposing biochemical force to arachidonic acid is the omega-3 family, which includes EPA (eicosapentaenoic acid) and DHA (docosahexaenoic acid).

These fatty acids compete with AA for COX and LOX enzymes, generating resolvins and protectins, both being molecules that *end* inflammation. By increasing dietary omega-3s from algae, flax, chia, and walnuts while eliminating dairy and meat, the AA: EPA ratio drops, and prostaglandin production normalizes.

Emotional Cleansing Through Chemistry

As inflammation recedes and the fog dissipates, emotional tone lifts and the chest opens. People describe the sensation as *"light returning to the blood."* This is a mitochondrial response.

Serotonin production rises, cortisol stabilizes, and the nervous system shifts from *fight and inflame* to *rest and regenerate*. The body learns that peace is our default state once the biochemical chaos of dairy is removed.

Nutrients that Calm the Flame

• **Curcumin** (from turmeric): blocks COX-2 enzyme activity as effectively as NSAIDs, without side effects.

• **Gingerols** (from ginger): inhibit prostaglandin biosynthesis and soothe digestion.

• **Boswellic acids** (from frankincense): reduce leukotriene formation.

• **Magnesium**: stabilizes cell membranes and lowers inflammatory cytokines.

• **Polyphenols** (from berries, cacao, and green tea): neutralize free radicals and regenerate antioxidants like glutathione.

These compounds work not by numbing symptoms but by restoring harmony to the inflammatory conversation.

Reflection

Arachidonic acid is ancient. This is a molecule that served us when survival meant constant alertness. Humanity's evolution now demands a new chemistry that is not one of fight, flight, and flame, but of flow, presence, and light. Dairy keeps us locked in the chemistry of conflict. To transcend is to evolve not only diet but destiny.

Chapter 10: The Hormonal Hijack

How Dairy Disrupts the Endocrine Symphony

There is a silent orchestra within every human being. Hormones are our musicians. They are minute, invisible, and infinitely precise. From a single drop of blood, they tune the entire symphony of life. This is displayed in our metabolism, mood, fertility, growth, and grace.

When we drink milk, however, we invite another creature's orchestra to play inside our own body. Unfortunately, the melodies do not harmonize. There can be instances where there is congruence for periods of time, but usually soon after there is an eruption and recognized incompatibility that warns us the band must break-up and our bodily sovereignty from foreign fluids is required.

Milk: A Hormonal Cocktail by Design

Every mammal's milk is a biological signal created for their offspring's stage of growth. Cow's milk contains estrogen, progesterone, cortisol, prolactin, growth hormone, and insulin-like growth factor-1 (IGF-1). Each of these are carefully balanced for the purpose of growing a 60-pound calf into a 600-pound animal within months.

Because modern dairy cows are milked during pregnancy, these hormones reach levels twenty to thirty times higher than in non-pregnant cows. Most are heat-stable steroids that survive processing and pasteurization intact. When human adults consume this fluid daily, they are not only ingesting fat and protein but are consuming a foreign endocrine system.

Estrogens and the Feminization of Humanity

Estrogens exist in several forms, including estrone (E1), estradiol (E2), and estriol (E3). In milk, the majority is estrone sulfate, which is a conjugated estrogen that remains active after digestion. Studies show that estrone sulfate passes through the intestinal wall and raises circulating estrogen levels measurably in both men and women.

For women, this additional estrogen feeds estrogen-dominant disorders such as fibroids, breast tenderness, endometriosis, and ovarian cysts. In men, this estrogen dampens testosterone synthesis, lowers sperm count, and increases fat deposition around the chest and abdomen.

In societies of high dairy intake, puberty arrives earlier, menopause is more symptomatic, and hormone-sensitive cancers flourish. The body's natural balance between androgenic and estrogenic forces tilts toward excess yin, which leads to softness, stagnation, and depletion of drive.

Progesterone and the Confused Cycle

Progesterone in milk, secreted in abundance during cow pregnancy, interacts with human progesterone receptors. In women already struggling with disrupted ovulatory cycles, the effect can be destabilizing, creating irregular menses and emotional volatility. In men, progesterone metabolites modulate GABA receptors in the brain, producing subtle sedation and mood flattening.

Over time, this *"borrowed calm"* becomes endocrine fatigue. This results from the hypothalamic-pituitary-gonadal axis slowing output because exogenous signals are already present. The body's music softens to silence.

Cortisol and the Stress Chemistry of Milk

Dairy also carries cortisol. This is the hormone of alertness and survival. The modern dairy cow, bred for relentless production, lives in chronic physiological stress. Her milk mirrors that biochemistry.

When humans consume this milk, the ingested cortisol and cortisol-like steroids subtly elevate basal cortisol levels, promoting chronic low-grade stress responses such as high blood pressure, abdominal fat storage, insomnia, and anxiety. The irony is sharp in that milk is marketed as comfort yet chemically reinforces distress.

IGF-1: Growth Without End

Among milk's most potent endocrine signals is insulin-like growth factor-1 (IGF-1), a peptide hormone identical in structure between cow and human. IGF-1 stimulates cellular proliferation and inhibits apoptosis, which is the programmed cell death that keeps tissues youthful and clean. Dairy consumption raises plasma IGF-1 by ten to twenty percent within weeks. While this may aid growth in children, in adults this fuels cancer progression, acne, polycystic ovarian syndrome (PCOS), and prostate hypertrophy.

IGF-1 also amplifies mTORC1, the cellular growth switch, locking the body into perpetual anabolic mode. When growth never pauses, regeneration never begins. The body becomes crowded with unchecked creation.

Prolactin and the Chemistry of Attachment

Milk naturally contains prolactin, the hormone of nurturing and bonding. In the infant-mother pair, prolactin reinforces love and trust. In adults who ingest milk daily, this neuro-endocrine signal lingers, blurring emotional independence.

Many people experience *"comfort"* in cheese or warm milk at night not from nutrition but from this molecular mimicry of maternal bonding. The experience can soothe the nervous system temporarily while weakening the natural dopamine tone that maintains autonomy and motivation. The same mechanism underlies addictive attachment to dairy's casomorphins, where there is chemical comfort disguised as counterfeit affection.

The Endocrine Web: Cascading Consequences

When foreign hormones enter, the body responds through feedback inhibition. The hypothalamus and pituitary sense the surplus and reduce their own production of gonadotropins, thyroid-stimulating hormone, and growth hormone.

This cascade produces measurable effects, which include:

• **Reduced thyroid output** → slower metabolism, cold extremities, fatigue.

• **Suppressed luteinizing hormone (LH)** → impaired ovulation and testosterone synthesis.

• **Increased prolactin** → menstrual irregularity, lowered libido, breast enlargement in men.

Over time, these imbalances manifest as what modern medicine calls *syndrome* rather than source, treating each symptom in isolation, and never tracing back to the milk.

Endocrine Disruption Across Generations

Exposure begins even before birth. Pregnant women consuming dairy transmit these bovine hormones across the placenta. Infants fed cow's-milk formula receive not only casein and lactose but an exogenous hormonal imprint during their most vulnerable phase of development.

Epidemiological data link early cow's-milk exposure to increased risk of juvenile diabetes, early puberty, and infantile acne. These are all markers of endocrine dysregulation. Thus, the hijack is hereditary.

Environmental Estrogens and the Feminized Planet

The issue extends beyond the body. Dairy effluent, that is laden with unmetabolized estrogens, flows into rivers, altering fish reproduction and contaminating groundwater. Scientists have detected feminized male fish downstream from dairy farms and municipal wastewater rich in steroid residues. Even the planet experiences endocrine confusion.

Healing the Endocrine Symphony

To restore balance, the first step is silence. We accomplish this with the removal of the foreign orchestra. When dairy leaves, the human endocrine system re-awakens. Within months, studies show reductions in circulating estrogen, normalization of testosterone, and improved insulin sensitivity.

Supportive nutrients for recalibration:

• **Cruciferous vegetables** (broccoli, kale, cabbage): contain indole-3-carbinol and sulforaphane, which assist estrogen detoxification through the liver.

• **Flaxseed and chia**: lignans modulate estrogen receptor activity naturally.

• **Zinc and selenium**: vital for testosterone synthesis and thyroid conversion.

• **Adaptogens** (ashwagandha, maca, rhodiola): rebuild the hypothalamic-pituitary balance.

• **Fiber and hydration**: ensure that liberated hormones exit through the colon instead of recirculating.

As hormones rebalance and clarity returns, sleep deepens, mood steadies, and libido rekindles. The body regains a rightful rhythm.

Reflection

To drink milk is to play another species' symphony inside the human instrument. The notes may sound soft at first, but the harmony collapses with time. The true nourishment of adulthood is not growth but equilibrium.

When we relinquish the hormones of the cow, we reclaim the intelligence of our own chemistry. In that quiet, the body remembers our original song.

Chapter 11: The Microbiome War

How Dairy Disrupts the Inner Garden of Life

There are more of them than there are of us. Trillions of bacteria, archaea, fungi, and viruses form an invisible ecosystem inside the human body. Visualize this as an inner rainforest that digests food, trains immunity, and even shapes emotion. Together, they are called the microbiome, and when in harmony, they generate the quiet electricity of health.

If we feed this rainforest the wrong substance, the once flowing ecosystem turns to stagnant swamp. Dairy is that wrong substance that fertilizes the microbes of decay and starves the microbes of light.

A Living Network Between Worlds

The gut is more of a forest floor than a pipe. Roughly 100 trillion microorganisms live in the folds, producing short-chain fatty acids (SCFAs) such as butyrate, acetate, and propionate. Each of these molecules are important and they lower inflammation, feed colon cells, and strengthen the intestinal barrier.

The microbiome also manufactures vitamins B and K, communicates with the brain via the vagus nerve, and calibrates immunity through dendritic cells along the intestinal wall. When this ecosystem is balanced, we feel clarity and calm. When poisoned by the wrong foods, especially the casein and fats of dairy, the ecosystem shifts into dysbiosis, assembling a microbial civil war.

Casein: The Colon's Glue

Casein, the dominant protein in milk, is difficult to hydrolyze. Incomplete digestion leaves behind bioactive peptides that resist further breakdown. These peptides stick to the intestinal lining, feeding mucus-eating bacteria such as *Akkermansia muciniphila* in excess, and allowing opportunists like *Clostridium perfringens*, *Proteus mirabilis*, and *E. coli* to flourish.

The result is putrefaction rather than fermentation. Instead of producing butyrate (which heals), these microbes produce ammonia, amines, hydrogen sulfide, and lipopolysaccharides (LPS), all of which irritate the intestinal wall and leak into the bloodstream. This *"metabolic endotoxemia"* quietly inflames every organ touched.

The Acid Terrain

Dairy digestion leaves an acidic residue, lowering colonic pH below optimal range for beneficial *Bifidobacteria* and *Lactobacilli*. An acidified gut favors yeast and sulfate-reducing bacteria that generate hydrogen sulfide gas. This is the source of bloating, bad breath, and brain fog. As acidity increases, the gut's electrical potential drops and nutrient absorption falters. The inner soil loses voltage.

Bacterial Endotoxins & Systemic Inflammation

Lipopolysaccharides from Gram-negative bacteria penetrate compromised intestinal junctions and activate Toll-Like Receptor 4 (TLR-4) on immune cells. This triggers the release of interleukin-6, tumor necrosis factor-α, and C-reactive protein, creating body-wide inflammation. These cytokines impair insulin signaling, dull the thyroid, and cross the blood–brain barrier to disturb mood and motivation.

Candida & the Sugar of Milk

Milk's lactose is a double sugar (glucose & galactose). When unabsorbed, this becomes fuel for Candida albicans and other yeasts. Antibiotics, stress, and low stomach acid compound the problem, leading to overgrowths that manifest as cravings, sinus congestion, fatigue, and recurring skin eruptions. Candida thrives where dairy residues linger and there is damp, acidic, and sweet.

The Gut–Brain Axis

Microbes manufacture neurotransmitters. *Lactobacillus* produces GABA, *Bifidobacterium* makes tryptophan for serotonin, and *Clostridium sporogenes* releases toxins that alter dopamine pathways. When dairy shifts the microbiome toward the latter, our mood often follows, resulting in more anxiety, irritability, and lethargy. Scientific studies confirm that LPS-induced inflammation alters brain function, creating what researchers call "sickness behavior." We see this displayed through social withdrawal, low motivation, and mental fog. The gut truly is the first brain and dairy muddies the messages being directed to us.

Immune Disarray

Seventy percent of the immune system lives in the gut-associated lymphoid tissue (GALT). Casein fragments cross the epithelial barrier and mimic human tissue sequences, provoking molecular mimicry and autoimmunity.

Conditions such as Hashimoto's thyroiditis, rheumatoid arthritis, and multiple sclerosis show improved outcomes when dairy is eliminated, suggesting that the immune confusion begins in the bowel.

The Raw Milk Myth

Some argue that *"raw milk"* supports beneficial bacteria. Yet microbial analyses reveal that unpasteurized milk often harbors *Listeria*, *Campylobacter*, *Salmonella*, and *E. coli O157:H7*. These are species capable of producing shiga toxins and endotoxins far more harmful than any probiotic benefit. Even in sterile laboratory settings, raw milk ferments into acid-forming by-products that destabilize gut pH. Living does not always mean life-giving.

Re-Cultivating the Inner Garden

When dairy disappears, the microbial terrain begins to rewild:

• Within days, pH normalizes and butyrate-producing species rebound.

• Within weeks, intestinal permeability improves; CRP and IL-6 decline.

• Within months, serotonin levels and cognitive clarity rise.

To aid this regeneration:

• **Prebiotics:** resistant starch and inulin from chicory, green bananas, and Jerusalem artichoke.

• **Probiotics:** plant-based fermented foods such as sauerkraut, kimchi, coconut kefir, or soy-free tempeh.

• **Polyphenols:** blueberries, cacao, and green tea provide these antioxidants that feed beneficial microbes.

• **Digestive cleansing:** colon hydrotherapy, herbal bitters, ozone, and hydration to flush residue.

The goal is not sterility but *symbiosis*. We pave a path to establish a peace treaty between human and microbe.

The Spiritual Dimension

The microbiome is more than biology. Each species holds fragments of ancient Earth. The same bacteria that once fixed nitrogen in soil now live in our intestines. When we poison them with alien fats and denatured proteins, we disrupt the covenant between human and planet. To heal the gut is to restore our conversation with the living world.

Reflection

Dairy turns the inner garden into a battleground. Remove this culprit, and the soil softens, the air returns, and the roots of vitality re-emerge. Every bowel movement becomes a prayer of purification, and each breath a renewal of symbiosis. The war ends not with antibiotics, but with abstinence and awareness.

Chapter 12: The Calcium Conspiracy

How the Dairy Industry Sold Weakness as Strength

From childhood, the story is poured into us as faithfully as the milk. A white glass on the breakfast table, with a smiling cartoon cow, and the slogan echoing through every school cafeteria: *"Milk builds strong bones."*

This is one of the most successful, and most damaging, marketing myths ever told. The truth, whispered quietly through decades of nutritional science, is the opposite: dairy's calcium *leaves* the bones rather than builds them. The arteries are hardened while the skeleton is hollowed. This is the great calcium conspiracy.

The Myth of the Milk Mineral

Calcium is indeed vital. This mineral composes the crystalline scaffolding of bones and teeth, enables muscle contraction, governs heartbeat rhythm, and stabilizes cellular membranes. The issue is not calcium, but the version of calcium we ingest with bovine milk, and the medium through which the compound is delivered.

In the 1950s, dairy marketing boards realized that *"protein for strength"* was no longer enough to justify mass consumption. So, they pivoted to calcium, recasting milk as a *"liquid bone."* Campaigns featuring athletes and celebrities turned a single nutrient into an industry shield, one strong enough to deflect all criticism.

The science, however, never supported the claims. Populations consuming the most milk, consisting of the United States, Finland, Sweden, and New Zealand, have consistently shown the highest rates of osteoporosis and hip fractures. Meanwhile, rural African and Asian populations with minimal dairy intake enjoy the strongest bones and lowest fracture rates in the world.

Acid-Ash & the Calcium Drain

Every food leaves behind a residue of minerals and metabolites that determine whether this is acid-forming or alkaline-forming in the body. Animal proteins like casein and whey metabolize into sulfuric and phosphoric acids, which must be neutralized to maintain blood pH at 7.345. The body achieves this by extracting calcium phosphate and magnesium from bones and teeth, using them as emergency buffers. In other words, each glass of milk may provide calcium, but the digestion process *steals* more than gives.

This is the biological sleight of hand behind dairy's illusion of strength. We have a food that gives calcium with one hand and takes other vital nutrients with the other.

Protein Overload & the Calcium Leak

The high protein load of dairy, especially casein, stimulates glomerular filtration in the kidneys and increases urinary calcium excretion. Even if dietary calcium intake rises, so does calcium loss. Imagine pouring water into a bucket while simultaneously drilling holes in the base. This is what dairy does to the bones. Calcium balance depends not on how much enters the mouth, but how much remains in the body, and the dairy equation is negative.

Phosphorus: The Bone Bandit

Dairy contains more phosphorus than calcium. While both minerals are essential, an excess of phosphorus increases parathyroid hormone (PTH) secretion, which draws calcium from bones to correct the blood ratio. High-P diets, especially from cheese and processed dairy, accelerate bone resorption, leading to porosity and fragility. This is why populations drowning in cheese often experience a high prevalence in osteoporosis as well.

Hormonal Chaos: IGF-1 and the Bone Matrix

Dairy's IGF-1 (Insulin-Like Growth Factor 1) temporarily increases bone formation by stimulating osteoblasts, but simultaneously elevates osteoclast activity, the cells that dissolve bone tissue. The net effect is *disorganization*, where bone turnover outpaces bone strength, leading to structurally weaker bones even if density appears stable. In short, dairy builds bulk but not integrity. You receive a scaffolding of chalk rather than stone.

Calcification: Hard Where We Should Be Soft

Excess calcium from dairy does not always lodge in bones. Often, this sludge precipitates in the wrong places, including the arteries, kidneys, joints, and glands. When combined with oxidized fats from homogenized milk, free calcium ions form calcium soaps and plaques that stiffen arteries and calcify soft tissue.

This phenomenon, known as ectopic calcification, is now recognized as a major factor in heart disease and Alzheimer's pathology. Calcium without cofactors like vitamin K2, magnesium, and boron is a wanderer without a map. The bones thin as the arteries harden.

Bone Health: The Alkaline Truth

True bone strength depends on mineral synergy:

• Magnesium directs calcium into bone tissue and prevents arterial calcification.

• Vitamin D facilitates calcium absorption but requires magnesium to activate.

• Vitamin K2 activates osteocalcin, the protein that locks calcium into bone.

• Silica, boron, and plant-based phytonutrients fortify collagen, which is the lattice on which minerals crystallize.

These cofactors abound not in milk, but in plants:

• Dark leafy greens, sesame seeds, figs, and almonds.

• Amaranth, quinoa, and tofu (if non-GMO and organic).

• Herbs like horsetail and nettle, rich in silica and boron.

When these foods dominate the diet, calcium finds a rightful home.

The pH of Purity

Bone health reflects systemic pH balance. When the body is alkaline, meaning rich in plant minerals, chlorophyll, and bicarbonate ions, calcium remains in storage, and bone density stabilizes. When the diet is acid-forming, or heavy with dairy, meat, sugar, and stress, calcium becomes the first responder to the fire, extinguishing acidity at the cost of structure. Thus, osteoporosis is not a calcium deficiency, but mineral mismanagement caused by dietary misinformation.

Marketing the Myth

The dairy industry has long manipulated public perception through government-funded programs like "Got Milk?" and school lunch mandates. In 1993, the U.S. National Dairy Council spent over $200 million lobbying for federal guidelines emphasizing milk as a *"core calcium source,"* despite growing evidence to the contrary.

When independent studies questioned the bone benefits of milk, industry-funded reviews quickly appeared to neutralize the headlines. This is narrative control, not nutrition. The *"calcium connection"* between milk and bones was never scientific.

The Global Picture

The correlation is clear that when more milk is consumed, there are significantly more fractures.

• In Africa, average calcium intake from plant sources is only 300 mg/day, yet fracture rates are 50–100 times lower than in dairy-rich nations.

• In Japan, where green vegetables and seaweeds are primary calcium sources, osteoporosis rates remain among the world's lowest despite minimal milk consumption.

• In the U.S., where daily calcium intake often exceeds 1,000 mg, largely from dairy, osteoporosis affects over ten million adults and leads to two million fractures annually.

Rebuilding the Human Skeleton

Bone regeneration is not a matter of more calcium, but about creating the conditions for mineral intelligence. Bones are not stones; they are living tissues that respond to every thought, meal, and emotion.

1. Alkalinity: Daily intake of raw greens, vegetable juices, and citrus minerals restores bicarbonate buffering capacity.

2. Movement: Weight-bearing exercise stimulates osteoblasts through piezoelectric signals. This is electricity created when bone is compressed.

3. Sunlight & Vitamin D: Enhances calcium absorption and strengthens immune function.

4. Magnesium & K2: Found in pumpkin seeds, cacao, leafy greens, and natto (fermented soybeans). These nutrients keep calcium mobile and intelligent.

5. Emotional Stability: Stress hormones, especially cortisol, dissolve bone over time. Meditation, breathwork, and exposure to nature are as crucial as diet in maintaining skeletal vitality.

Jacoby/Lowther

Reflection

The calcium conspiracy is a story of misplaced trust. There is unwavering faith in advertising over anatomy. Milk was never meant to build human bones. This formula was designed to build hooves. Strength is not in the whiteness of a liquid, but in the clarity of truth.

The day we stop pouring another species' milk into our bodies is the day our bones stop crumbling under the weight of illusion.

Chapter 13: Healing Beyond the Herd

Reclaiming the Body's Sacred Intelligence

To stop drinking milk is an act of liberation. You make the choice to return from imitation nourishment to authentic life. For decades, humanity has sought vitality through the chemistry of another creature, the cow, believing that strength, fertility, and comfort could be borrowed, but this belief has chained our biology to stagnation.

When dairy finally leaves, our body begins to remember our original design. The rivers clear, lymph stirs, gut breathes, and a symphony of cellular repair begins to play.

The Body's Memory of Wholeness

The human organism is a living archive of purity. Every organ holds the memory of how to function in balance, yet that memory becomes muffled beneath years of chemical noise. Once dairy is removed, the first sensation many feel is *quiet*. This is not deprivation, but absence of interference. This quiet is the experience of intelligence returning.

The endocrine system resumes rhythm, microbiome rewilds, blood's pH stabilizes, and mitochondria begin generating current instead of fatigue. Science calls this "homeostasis."

Stage 1: The Purge: Lymphatic Awakening

The first weeks of detoxification can feel like a reckoning. The lymphatic system, which has spent years thickened by mucoproteins and oxidized fats, begins to drain. Mucus moves, bowels loosen, skin erupts, and sinuses release. This is not sickness you are experiencing, but rather is excretion. The body begins pulling long-stored waste from the reservoirs.

Support the purge:

• Hydrate with three to four liters daily of structured, mineralized water.

• Movement, including a rebounder, yoga twists, dry brushing, sauna, and breathwork to pump lymph.

• Colon hydrotherapy or enemas to flush lower channels.

• Bitters and bile stimulants such as dandelion root, milk thistle, lemon, and ginger.

Within two to three weeks, heaviness lifts, breath deepens, and the skin brightens. These are all signs that lymph and blood are communicating again.

Stage 2: The Rebuild: Microbiome Renewal

With the burden removed, the inner terrain reclaims balance. Beneficial bacteria such as *Lactobacillus plantarum*, *Bifidobacterium longum*, and *Faecalibacterium prausnitzii* recolonize the colon, producing butyrate. This is the molecule of intestinal peace. Butyrate nourishes colonocytes, reduces inflammation, and seals leaky junctions.

To accelerate this regeneration:

• **Prebiotic fibers:** Jerusalem artichoke, green bananas, leeks, chicory root, and acacia fiber.

• **Fermented plants:** sauerkraut, kimchi, coconut kefir, and beet kvass.

• **Polyphenol-rich fruits:** blueberries, pomegranate, cacao, and green tea are antioxidants that feed beneficial microbes.

• **Digestive enzymes:** bromelain, papain, and lipase assist in breaking down residual dairy deposits.

In four to six weeks, gut permeability improves measurably, cytokine levels drop, and serotonin synthesis increases. This lightens the mood.

Stage 3: The Rewire: Endocrine Recalibration

After years of ingesting bovine estrogens and growth factors, the endocrine orchestra requires retuning. The pituitary, thyroid, and adrenal glands begin to find their rhythm again once exogenous hormones are gone.

Restoration comes through minerals and adaptogens:

• **Zinc** (pumpkin seeds, spirulina, cacao) restores testosterone and thyroid hormone conversion.

• **Iodine** (seaweed, kelp) supports thyroid function and detoxifies halides stored in glandular tissue.

• **Ashwagandha** and **maca** stabilize cortisol and reproductive hormones.

• **Cruciferous vegetables** (broccoli, kale, mustard greens) promote estrogen metabolism via the liver's cytochrome P450 enzymes.

The hormonal clarity that follows is profound. Energy steadies, libido awakens, and emotional balance returns. You begin to feel *clean power* instead of stimulation.

Stage 4: The Ascension: Bioelectrical Renewal

When blood becomes alkaline and lymph moves freely, a new level of vitality emerges — a sensation of current. The body is not merely chemical; it is electrical. Each cell maintains a **membrane potential** of roughly -70 millivolts, powered by minerals and light.

Dairy's acid-forming residue once drained that voltage, forcing mitochondria to work harder. Now, voltage is restored.

Enhance cellular electricity through:

• **Sunlight exposure:** stimulates mitochondrial photoreceptors (cytochrome c oxidase) and boosts ATP.

• **Barefoot grounding:** recharges antioxidant potential through free electron exchange with Earth.

• **Deep breathing:** increases oxygen tension & redox potential.

• **Raw fruits and green juices:** carry structured water and bio-photons. This is light encoded in living molecules.

The result is heightened perception. You *feel* your cells glowing, like a quiet hum under the skin that science cannot yet quantify, but consciousness recognizes as aliveness.

Liver & Gallbladder Liberation

The liver, having filtered dairy's fats and hormones for years, finally exhales. The bile thins, enzymes normalize, and detoxification pathways reopen. Increased production of glutathione, the body's master antioxidant, restores cellular repair.

Supportive allies:

• Milk thistle (silymarin) regenerates hepatocytes.

• Artichoke leaf enhances bile flow.

• Turmeric and black pepper reduce hepatic inflammation.

• Castor oil packs over the liver area mobilize stagnant bile and lymph.

When the liver is clean, the eyes whiten, skin clears, and mood stabilizes. This is proof that purification and perception are linked.

Emotional Detox: The Chemistry of Release

Dairy binds emotionally as much as biochemically. The casomorphins mimic opioids and prolactin mimics maternal comfort. When these compounds leave the system, old emotions often rise to the surface. We experience these as grief, craving, loneliness, and nostalgia.

These are not just memories of taste but of identity. We can often feel the loss of *"comfort food"* associated with childhood and safety.

To move through this:

• Breathe deeply when cravings hit. Oxygen dissolves emotional chemistry.

• Hydrate, as water dilutes the biochemical memory of craving.

• Journal or meditate, let buried emotions speak and pass.

Within this emotional clearing lies true freedom and nourishment without dependency.

Spiritual Integration: From Herd to Heart

The deeper liberation from dairy is symbolic. The cow represents domestication and a gentleness bound to servitude. Humanity's dependence on her milk mirrors our dependence on comfort over consciousness.

To step beyond dairy is to step beyond domestication and return to wild purity. We go back to living n a way that is guided not by advertising or addiction, but by intuition. The *"herd"* is both literal and psychological. This represents the social conditioning that says we need what weakens us.

When one human remembers otherwise, the herd begins to heal.

Sustaining the Cleansed State

After detox, maintenance becomes devotion. In this lifestyle, the body no longer seeks external comfort but radiates internal light.

• **Daily rhythm:** early rising, movement, hydration, and mindful meals.

• **Periodic fasting:** one day per week or seasonal three-day juice fasts for cellular reset.

• **Continued alkalinity:** eighty percent plant-based raw diet with seasonal fruits and greens.

• **Gratitude:** conscious appreciation re-entrains the nervous system toward peace and is the ultimate antidote to inflammation.

Reflection

The end of dairy is a deliverance and reclamation of the body's right to vibrate at our natural frequency in a way that is uncoated, undiluted, and awake.

When the milk of another species leaves the bloodstream, the milk of human kindness begins to flow again. This rediscovered compassion is not compelled by addiction but born from clarity. Healing beyond the herd is healing into humanity.

Epilogue: Returning to Purity

Healing the Body, Healing the Earth

The story of milk is the story of forgetfulness. Once, every species knew their own rhythm, nursed their young, and then weaned, moving from dependency to self-sustaining wisdom. Somewhere along humanity's climb toward civilization, we stopped weaning. We turned backward, not to nature but to the udder of another creature, and we built an empire on that dependency.

For centuries, milk has been more than a beverage. This has been symbol and sacrament of a cultural emblem of purity that concealed the opposite. In the name of nourishment, we learned to consume what numbs us, and in the name of comfort, we learned to silence discomfort rather than learn. Now the veil lifts.

The Great Remembering

To stop drinking milk is not to reject the cow but is to release the illusion that we need her chemistry to complete our own. We honor her as a fellow being, not a vessel. We break the ancestral trance that equates comfort with sedation, and nourishment with addiction.

When we return to our natural diet, consisting of fruits that shimmer with sunlight, greens that hum with minerals, and waters that carry the memory of mountains, we participate in the great remembering. This is the restoration of alignment between species, elements, and consciousness.

Health is not a supplement or a food group, but is relationship between body and soil, breath and tree, and human and planet.

Purity as a Frequency

Purity is the absence of distortion in the body's communication with life. When our fluids run clear, our thoughts follow. When lymph flows, emotion flows. When oxygen saturates the blood, clarity saturates the mind.

This purity radiates outward. Clean people create clean choices. This is indicated in clean energy, clean soil, and clean water. In this way, each act of personal detoxification becomes planetary healing. The dairy detox is a spiritual ecology and reminds us that the body and Earth share one bloodstream.

The End of Flesh, The Beginning of Life

The end of dairy marks more than the removal of a food; this is also the end of a worldview that says survival requires subjugation. When we stop consuming the secretions of another, we stop consuming the suffering that produced them. We stop ingesting the chemistry of confinement, fear, and hormonal confusion that defines industrial life.

What begins in the bloodstream becomes revolution in the psyche. As the body purifies, perception changes. We see through the advertising fog, governmental half-truths, and medical dogma, all of which, like casein, were built to bind.

As the fog lifts, so does fatigue. Energy returns. Compassion expands. Life feels alive again. The end of flesh is not death but is an awakening, and a return to the living foods that carry sunlight rather than suffering.

The Planetary Parallel

The planet, too, is clearing her mucus. Oceans foam with industrial runoff, rivers choke on the residue of agriculture, and skies exhale smoke like congested lungs. Humanity's relationship with dairy mirrors our relationship with the Earth. There is extraction disguised as nourishment, and dependence disguised as care.

When we purify our own bodies, we break the mirror of exploitation. Each plant-based meal is a prayer for the rivers, and every clear breath an act of restoration. Healing the human bloodstream heals the planetary bloodstream; both are one continuum of circulation and consciousness.

A New Kind of Strength

True strength is not in milk-fed muscle but in mineral-fed mind. We experience this as the quiet confidence that arises when we know our vitality is clean and has been earned through truth rather than advertising. In the courage to let go of cultural comfort and trust nature's original design. To live milk-free is to live myth-free. To live myth-free is to live awake. The awake human, clear of mucus, free of addiction, and radiant with oxygen and purpose, is the seed of a new civilization.

Closing Benediction

May your blood run clear. May your breath flow unhindered. May your bones be light and strong, your skin translucent, and your eyes bright with voltage. May your compassion extend to all species, including your own. Additionally, may your life become the living proof that purity is power, health is clarity, and the end of dependency is the beginning of divinity.

Author's Note: From Addiction to Alignment

There was a time when I believed what the billboards said. That milk was strength. That cheese was comfort. That a white glass at breakfast meant health.

The truth had been inverted, though, and I learned that the very thing sold as vitality was the slow erosion. When I stopped consuming dairy, the body I thought was "normal" was revealed as burdened. The sinuses that had always been clogged, the skin that occasionally broke out, and the afternoon fatigue I thought was just life all dissolved within weeks.

My realization was not simply that I felt better but that I started to feel awake, clearer, cleaner, and connected. For the first time, I could feel my lymph move when I breathed deeply. I could taste the sweetness of fruit the way a child does. Colors looked brighter and sound seemed closer. I felt as if an old fog had lifted, one that I had not known existed because I had been born inside of this density.

Fifteen Years of Purity

For fifteen years I have lived free from meat, dairy, alcohol, and pharmaceuticals. My journey has been part science, part spirit, and part rebellion. In that time, I have seen the body transform beyond what textbooks claim possible. I witnessed diseases reverse, hormones balance, addictions dissolve, and energy rise like a tide that never recedes. When we stop feeding the body confusion, the response is that the body illuminates.

As I worked with clients through detoxification, breathwork, ozone therapy, colon hydrotherapy, and nutritional re-education, I witnessed the same pattern repeat. When dairy was removed, the light returned. Eyes brightened, breath deepened, and mood stabilized.

The Scientific and the Sacred

Every chapter of this book bridges two worlds: the scientific and the sacred. Science offers the language of pathways through IGF-1, mTOR, LPS, cytokines, mitochondria. Spirit offers the language of pattern in stagnation and flow, suffocation and clarity, and bondage and release. Together they tell one story, that life either circulates or coagulates.

The chemistry of dairy is the chemistry of coagulation, not only in the blood, but in consciousness. This book is not written to condemn the cow, as she is a teacher. Her milk shows us what happens when we ignore natural law and is a mirror for our cultural dependency on stimulation, sedation, and false security. To heal, we must honor her by ending the exploitation of her motherhood and the theft of her chemistry.

Why We Wrote This Book

We wrote *Dirty Dairy* to lift the veil on one of the most normalized addictions in human history and to offer liberation through understanding. This book is the distillation of years of research, teaching, and observation from cellular biology to spiritual ecology.

These pages are both exposé and invitation. An exposé of an industry that markets mucus as medicine, and an invitation to return to the pure current of human design.

We believe that the human body is a divine technology capable of self-repair, illumination, and longevity far beyond current expectation. This technology cannot operate on distortion. To evolve, we must refine our inputs. We must eat for clarity, breathe for energy, and live for reverence.

A Final Word

You will not need milk once you begin to remember light. The minerals of the earth, the chlorophyll of leaves, the sap of fruit, and the structured water of living plants will become your new bloodstream.

When that happens, you will understand what we mean when we say that purity is power. We do not write of this as fragility or perfectionism but as electrical coherence. The purity we represent is the alignment of thought, body, and nature into one frequency.

May this book help you release what never belonged in you, and may your clarity become contagious.

Appendices

Appendix A: Dairy-Free Rebuilding Protocols

Restoring the Body's Flow After the Fog

When dairy leaves, the rivers in our body begin to move again, and the systems of detoxification awaken. These rebuilding protocols guide that renewal phase, restoring enzymatic function, lymphatic rhythm, and cellular vitality.

1. Morning Hydration & Alkaline Activation

• One-liter warm water with half lemon and a pinch of sea salt and trace minerals.

Purpose: stimulates bile flow, hydrates fascia, and begins daily alkalinity.

• Optional: add chlorophyll drops or fresh wheatgrass juice to oxygenate blood.

2. Lymphatic Movement

• Rebounding or brisk walking (ten to twenty minutes) upon waking.

• Dry brushing toward the heart before showering.

• Finish with contrast therapy (hot/cold alternation) to pump lymph.

3. Midday Cleansing Support

• Raw vegetable juice (celery, cucumber, parsley, fennel, lemon).

• Digestive enzyme complex with meals to assist protein breakdown.

• Avoid combining starches and fats in the same meal; simplify digestion to reduce mucus formation.

4. Evening Detox & Renewal

• Infrared sauna or Epsom-salt bath three to four times per week to mobilize waste through skin.

• Castor-oil pack over liver and gallbladder for forty-five minutes to thin bile.

• Breathwork or meditation before bed to activate parasympathetic repair.

5. Weekly Practices

• One liquid or fruit-based fasting day weekly (coconut water, green juice, herbal teas).

• Colon hydrotherapy or herbal bowel cleanse monthly during transition.

• Grounding barefoot in soil or sand to restore electromagnetic balance.

Appendix B: Recommended Supplements & Herbs for Detox

Catalysts of Cleansing and Cellular Renewal

Digestive & Systemic Enzymes

• *Protease, bromelain, papain, serrapeptase:* dissolve mucoproteins and scar tissue.

• *Lipase & amylase:* restore metabolic fire for fat and carbohydrate digestion.

Probiotics & Prebiotics

• Multi-strain Lactobacillus, Bifidobacterium, Bacillus Subtilus and other soil-based organisms (10–50 billion CFU daily).

• Feed with prebiotic fibers: inulin, acacia, Jerusalem artichoke, green bananas.

Herbal Detoxifiers

• *Milk thistle (silymarin):* liver regeneration.

• *Dandelion root & burdock:* lymphatic and hepatic drainage.

• *Ginger, turmeric, cayenne:* anti-inflammatory circulation boosters.

• *Schisandra & holy basil:* adaptogens for stress and oxidative protection.

Binders & Chelators

• *Activated charcoal or chlorella:* bind endotoxins & metals.

• *Zeolite & bentonite clay:* absorb metabolic acids.

• *Cilantro & parsley:* mobilize stored toxins from tissues.

Mineral Replenishment

• Magnesium glycinate or malate (300–400 mg / day).

• *Trace minerals:* fulvic acid, shilajit, or sea-mineral concentrates.

• *Iodine (kelp or nascent forms):* thyroid and lymphatic cleansing.

Optional Advanced Therapies (under guidance)

• Ozone insufflation or sauna.

• Hyperbaric oxygen.

• Infrared light therapy.

Appendix C: Plant-Based Calcium, Protein & Omega Sources

Building Strength from Light, Not from Flesh

Calcium Sources

• *Sesame seeds / tahini:* 120 mg per Tbsp.

• *Almonds:* 80 mg per oz.

• *Kale, bok choy, collards:* 90–150 mg per cup cooked.

• *Figs:* 60 mg per 4 figs.

• *Amaranth & quinoa:* 80 mg per cup cooked.

• *Blackstrap molasses:* 200 mg per Tbsp.

• *Mineral water rich in bicarbonate:* 50–100 mg per glass.

• *Enhancers:* vitamin D (sunlight), magnesium, vitamin K_2 (from natto or fermented foods), and silica (horsetail, cucumbers).

Protein Sources

• *Sprouted legumes/seeds (mung, lentil, chickpea):* 20–25 g per cup.

• *Hemp seeds:* 10 g per 3 Tbsp.

• *Chlorella & spirulina:* 60–70 % protein by weight & chlorophyll & B-vitamins.

• *Pumfu or soy-free Tempeh* (organic, non-GMO).

• *Pumpkin & sunflower seeds:* high zinc, immune support.

• *Quinoa / amaranth:* complete amino acid profiles.

• *Synergy:* combine pulses, grains, and greens for full amino balance without acid load.

Omega-3 & Anti-Inflammatory Fats

• *Flaxseed (ground):* rich in ALA.

• *Chia seeds:* balance omega-3 with omega-6.

• *Walnuts:* brain & vessel health.

• *Algal oil:* direct source of DHA / EPA.

• *Avocado:* monounsaturated fats for hormone regulation.

• *Perilla & purslane:* plant sources of omega-3 and antioxidants.

These fats stabilize cell membranes, enhance neurotransmission, and replace the inflammatory arachidonic acid found in animal dairy.

Appendix D: Key Scientific References & Influences

For the Reader Who Seeks Proof and Perspective

Foundational Texts

• Campbell, T. Colin & Campbell II, Thomas M. *The China Study*. BenBella Books, 2006.

• Warburg, Otto. *The Metabolism of Tumours*. Richard R. Smith, 1931.

• Nestle, Marion. *Food Politics: How the Food Industry Influences Nutrition and Health*. University of California Press, 2007.

• Hotema, Hilton. *Man's Higher Consciousness*. Health Research Books, 1952.

• Pizzorno, Joseph, et al. *Textbook of Natural Medicine*. 5th ed., Elsevier, 2020.

Peer-Reviewed Sources (NIH / PubMed)

• Melnik, B. C. "Milk signaling through mTORC1: a mechanism explaining common diseases of civilization." *Nutrients* 5 (2013): 1034–1061.

• Qin, L. Q. et al. "Milk consumption and circulating IGF-1 levels: systematic review." *Eur J Clin Nutr* 64 (2010): 1331–1339.

• Cani, P. D. & Delzenne, N. M. "The role of the gut microbiota in energy metabolism and metabolic disease." *Curr Pharm Des* 15 (2009): 1546–1558.

• Nedergaard, M. et al. "The glymphatic system: a waste-clearance system in the brain." *Science* 340 (2013): 1529–1531.

• Ridker, P. M. et al. "C-reactive protein and other markers of inflammation in CVD prediction." *NEJM* 347 (2002): 1557–1565.

• Sun, Z. & Cade, J. R. "A peptide found in schizophrenia and autism causes behavioral changes in rats." *Autism* 3 (1999): 85–95.

Philosophical & Spiritual Influences

• Thich Nhat Hanh – *Peace Is Every Step*

• Richard Rudd – *Gene Keys*

• Robin Wall Kimmerer – *Braiding Sweetgrass*

• Viktor Schauberger – *The Water Wizard*

• Hilton Hotema – *Sun and Earth Teachings of Light*

Closing Note

These appendices are blueprints, not afterthoughts. Knowledge without practice is theory, and practice without purity is exhaustion. The protocols, herbs, and foods within these pages are devised from the same principles that built this book. These include clarity over comfort, flow over fixation, and truth over tradition.

May they serve as living medicine and tools to help the reader transform information into illumination.

About the Authors

Jesse Jacoby is a dedicated father, expressionist, and advocate for compassion, equanimity, and purity. He expends energy adventuring in forests, creating, learning, playing, and writing. He has been following an all organic, fully plant-based, grain-free and alcohol-free lifestyle for fifteen years.

Jesse is the founder and CEO of Soulspire: The Healing Playground (*soulspire.com*). This is a biohacking and purification center with locations near Lake Tahoe in Truckee, CA, and in Nevada City, CA.

Jesse is the author of The Raw Cure: Healing Beyond Medicine (1st & 2nd Editions), The Way Knows, The Meat Effect, Dirty Dairy, You Are Not Powerless, Sovereign Biology, The Frequency Diet, Eating Plant-Based, and several other nonfiction titles. He and his children have also co-authored several kids' books implementing values and raising awareness around compassion and mindfulness.

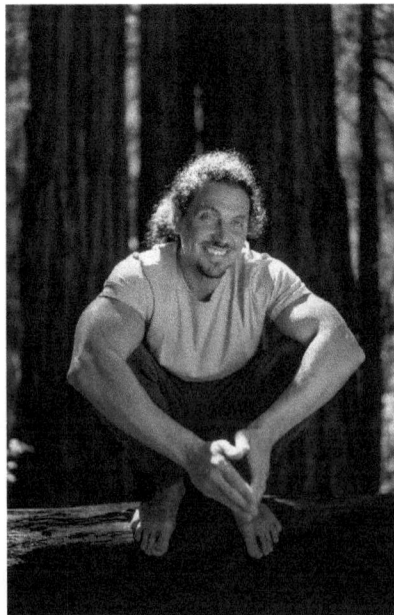

About the Authors

Born in Newcastle, UK, and now 45 years into a life defined by curiosity and evolution, Anthony Lowther has spent nearly three decades exploring the frontiers of human health. His journey from committed carnivore to devoted vegan, and from experimenter to embodiment reflects a rare level of rigor, humility, and lived inquiry.

Since the age of sixteen, Anthony has treated his body as a living laboratory, testing hypotheses, tracking outcomes, and observing how food becomes chemistry, chemistry becomes energy, and energy becomes the quality of a human life. For thirty years he explored the effects of a meat-heavy diet with scientific precision, then fifteen years ago pivoted into veganism with the same disciplined curiosity. His transition was a conscious choice rooted in ethics, physiology, and a deepening sense of responsibility to all living beings.

Anthony's work sits at the intersection of science, compassion, and systemic thinking. He is a practitioner who translates research into practical daily habits, a scientist who measures outcomes rather than opinions, and an advocate for a world in which human health and planetary health are no longer at odds. His guiding philosophy is simple yet profound, teaching that what sustains us must nourish all life, including humans, animals, and the ecosystems that hold us.

As a global community leader, Anthony has facilitated hundreds of retreats around the world, cultivating transformation for groups ranging from intimate circles of fifteen to celebratory gatherings of three hundred. He is also the founder of RISE & SHINE, a sober celebration platform where clarity, presence, and joy replace the distractions of modern culture.

Anthony's ambition is as bold as sincere. He aims to help create a system that works for all life while continually becoming the healthiest, most compassionate version of himself. His evolution is ongoing, measured weekly, lived fully, and shared openly. His life's work is a testament to continuous refinement, expanding consciousness, and an unwavering commitment to peace, vitality, and systemic harmony.

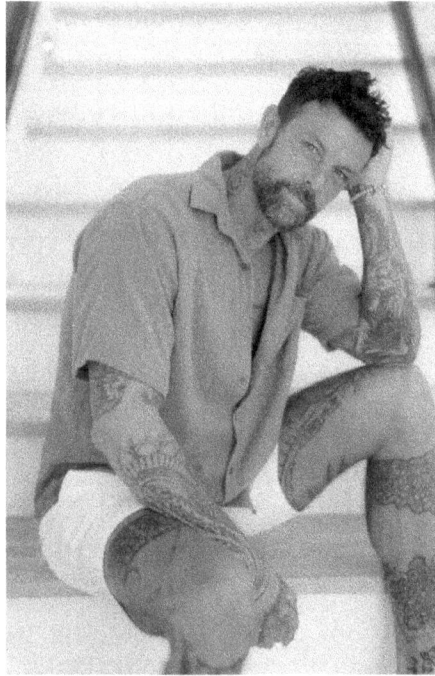

Bibliography

Chapter 1

• Wal, J.-M. "Bovine milk allergenicity and its clinical relevance." *Clinical Reviews in Allergy & Immunology* 30 (2006): 131–145.

• Blackburn, E. H., & Epel, E. S. "Telomeres and adversity: too much stress and unhealthy foods accelerate cellular aging." *Nature Reviews Immunology* 12 (2012): 467–473.

• Lerner, A., & Matthias, T. "Molecular mimicry mechanisms in food intolerance and autoimmunity." *Autoimmunity Reviews* 14 (2015): 479–489.

• Melnik, B. C. "Milk signaling through mTORC1: a mechanism explaining common diseases of civilization." *Nutrients* 5 (2013): 1034–1061.

• Abelow, B. J., Holford, T. R., & Insogna, K. L. "Cross-cultural association between dietary animal protein and hip fracture." *Calcified Tissue International* 50 (1992): 14–18.

• Barzel, U. S., & Massey, L. K. "Excess dietary protein can adversely affect bone." *Journal of Nutrition* 128 (1998): 1051–1053.

• Weaver, C. M. "Calcium nutrition and metabolism." *American Journal of Clinical Nutrition* 85 (2007): 1256S–1260S.

• Itan, Y. et al. "The origins of lactase persistence in Europe." *PLoS Computational Biology* 5 (2009): e1000491.

• Fasano, A. "Zonulin and its regulation of intestinal barrier function: the biological door to inflammation." *Physiological Reviews* 91 (2011): 151–175.

• Cani, P. D., & Delzenne, N. M. "The role of the gut microbiota in energy metabolism and metabolic disease." *Current Pharmaceutical Design* 15 (2009): 1546–1558.

Chapter 2

• Ahotupa, Markku. "Oxidized Lipoproteins and Atherosclerosis." *Free Radical Research*, vol. 51, no. 4, 2017, pp. 439–447.

• Aro, A., et al. "Dairy Fat and Coronary Heart Disease: Lipid Oxidation and LDL Damage." *American Journal of Clinical Nutrition*, vol. 65, no. 5, 1997, pp. 1410–1416.

• Bastida, Silvia, et al. "Lipid Oxidation and Oxysterol Formation in Heated Dairy Fats." *Journal of Agricultural and Food Chemistry*, vol. 47, no. 2, 1999, pp. 683–689.

• Bendtsen, Line Q., et al. "Dairy Fat, Plasma Lipids, and Inflammation." *American Journal of Clinical Nutrition*, vol. 99, no. 4, 2014, pp. 773–781.

• Bhat, Zuhaib F., et al. "Heterocyclic Amines in Cooked Meat and Fats: Chemistry and Toxicity." *Food Chemistry*, vol. 141, no. 3, 2013, pp. 389–399. (Relevant for ghee + animal fat frying.)

• Björck, Inger, et al. "Bioactive Components in Dairy and Their Health Effects." *Journal of Dairy Science*, vol. 94, no. 12, 2011, pp. 4743–4756. (Used for hormones, contaminants, and bioaccumulation.)

• Brenna, Øyvind, and Hilde G. Toft. "Thermal Oxidation of Cholesterol in Ghee." *International Dairy Journal*, vol. 17, no. 11, 2007, pp. 1251–1257.

• Carvalho, Leandro S., and Roberta F. S. Gonçalves. "Cholesterol Oxidation Products: Formation and Biological Effects." *Archives of Biochemistry and Biophysics*, vol. 707, 2022, 109002.

• Choe, Eunok, and David B. Min. "Chemistry of Deep-Fat Frying and Lipid Oxidation." *Journal of Food Science*, vol. 72, no. 5, 2007, pp. R77–R86.

• Delgado, L. C., and R. M. Gómez. "Oxidative Stress and Endothelial Injury from Dietary Cholesterol." *Biochimica et Biophysica Acta*, vol. 1851, no. 2, 2015, pp. 125–134.

• Esterbauer, Helmuth, et al. "Lipid Peroxidation and Oxidatively Modified LDL." *Free Radical Biology and Medicine*, vol. 13, no. 4, 1992, pp. 341–390.

• Fernandes, Paula A., et al. "Advanced Lipid Oxidation End Products and Their Impact on Health." *Journal of Nutritional Biochemistry*, vol. 25, no. 3, 2014, pp. 177–187.

• García-Linares, María C., et al. "Maillard Reaction Products in Heated Dairy Foods." *Food Chemistry*, vol. 130, no. 3, 2012, pp. 673–681.

• Gómez-Cortés, Pilar, et al. "Oxidative Stability of Milk Fat and Butter During Heating." *LWT – Food Science and Technology*, vol. 67, 2016, pp. 69–76.

• Hernandez, Elizabeth M., et al. "Thermal Effects on Lipopolysaccharides and Endotoxin Activity in Fat." *Journal of Food Protection*, vol. 62, no. 2, 1999, pp. 146–152.

• Hu, Frank B., et al. "Dairy Fat Intake and Risk of Cardiovascular Disease." *Circulation*, vol. 113, no. 16, 2006, pp. 2478–2487.

• Iqbal, Samina, et al. "Dioxins and PCBs in Dairy Products: Risk and Accumulation in Animal Fat." *Environmental Science and Pollution Research*, vol. 28, 2021, pp. 6769–6779.

• Jacobsen, Charlotte, et al. "Formation of Toxic Aldehydes During Heating of Animal Fats." *European Journal of Lipid Science and Technology*, vol. 109, no. 3, 2007, pp. 249–260.

• Kanner, Joseph, et al. "Dietary Fats and Oxidative Stress in the Human Body." *Critical Reviews in Food Science and Nutrition*, vol. 36, no. 4, 1996, pp. 313–327.

• Kolanowski, Wojciech, et al. "Environmental Contaminants in Butter and Ghee." *Food Control*, vol. 12, 2001, pp. 121–128.

• Liu, X., et al. "Oxysterols: From Cholesterol Metabolites to Key Mediators." *Journal of Lipid Research*, vol. 59, no. 8, 2018, pp. 1272–1285.

• Napoli, Claudio, et al. "Lipid Peroxidation, Antioxidant Depletion, and Endothelial Dysfunction." *Atherosclerosis*, vol. 161, no. 2, 2002, pp. 435–446.

• Niki, Etsuo. "Lipid Oxidation and Health Effects." *Free Radical Biology and Medicine*, vol. 44, no. 7, 2008, pp. 1116–1123.

• Papuc, Costin, et al. "Mechanisms of Oxidative Processes in Meat and Dairy Fats." *Comprehensive Reviews in Food Science and Food Safety*, vol. 16, no. 3, 2017, pp. 415–436.

• Sampaio, Guilherme R., et al. "Formation of Cholesterol Oxidation Products in Heated Foods." *Food Chemistry*, vol. 149, 2014, pp. 388–393.

• Seiquer, Irene, et al. "Oxidized Fats Produce Oxidative Stress and Endothelial Dysfunction in Humans." *Journal of Nutrition*, vol. 138, no. 1, 2008, pp. 36–41.

• Simopoulos, Artemis P. "Saturated Fat, Cholesterol, and Chronic Disease." *Journal of the American College of Nutrition*, vol. 21, no. 4, 2002, pp. 287–293.

• Smith, Kelly R., et al. "Inhalation of Cooking Vapors: Aldehydes and Carcinogens in Heated Animal Fats." *Environmental Research*, vol. 132, 2014, pp. 236–241.

• Török, Zsolt, et al. "Membrane Damage from Lipid Oxidation." *Progress in Lipid Research*, vol. 51, no. 2, 2012, pp. 122–152.

• Vasavada, Pratibha C., et al. "Formation of Oxysterols and Other Oxidized Lipids During Heating of Butter." *Journal of Food Science*, vol. 66, no. 6, 2001, pp. 817–822.

• Wyss, Michael T., et al. "Blood Flow, Endothelial Function, and Mitochondrial Efficiency Under Oxidative Stress." *Nature Reviews Neuroscience*, vol. 19, 2018, pp. 185–197.

Chapter 3

• Brantl, V. et al. "Opioid activities of β-casomorphins." *Life Sciences* 28 (1981): 1903–1909.

• Holzer, P. "Neural regulation of gastrointestinal motility by peptides." *Physiological Reviews* 69 (1989): 967–1023.

• Cani, P. D. et al. "Metabolic endotoxemia initiates obesity and insulin resistance." *Diabetes* 56 (2007): 1761–1772.

• Panksepp, J. "Affective neuroscience of social emotions and attachment." *Neuroscience & Biobehavioral Reviews* 23 (1999): 555–579.

• Sokolov, O. et al. "β-Casomorphin-7 in autism spectrum disorder." *Nutrients* 6 (2014): 875–886.

• McCarthy, D. O. et al. "Opioid peptides and immune function." *Advances in Neuroimmunology* 4 (1994): 191–198.

• Drewnowski, A. "Fat and sugar: an addictive combination." *American Journal of Clinical Nutrition* 62 (1995): 1081S–1085S.

• Sun, Z., & Cade, J. R. "A peptide found in schizophrenia and autism causes behavioral changes in rats." *Autism* 3 (1999): 85–95.

• Dandekar, S. P. et al. "β-Casomorphin's effects on catecholamine metabolism." *Journal of Neurochemistry* 55 (1990): 2169–2174.

•Barnard, N. D. et al. "Dietary intervention alters mood and productivity." *American Journal of Health Promotion* 32 (2018): 795–803.

Chapter 4

- Campbell, T. Colin, & Campbell, Thomas M. *The China Study*. BenBella Books, 2006.
- Qin, L. Q., et al. "Milk consumption and circulating insulin-like growth factor-I level: a systematic literature review." *European Journal of Clinical Nutrition* 64.12 (2010): 1331–1339.
- Melnik, B. C. "Milk signaling through mTORC1: a mechanism explaining common diseases of civilization." *Nutrients* 5 (2013): 1034–1061.
- Rowlands, M. A., et al. "Circulating insulin-like growth factor peptides and prostate cancer risk." *International Journal of Cancer* 124.10 (2009): 2416–2422.
- Renehan, A. G., et al. "Insulin-like growth factor (IGF)-I, IGF-binding protein-3, and cancer risk: systematic review and meta-regression analysis." *The Lancet* 363.9418 (2004): 1346–1353.
- Ganmaa, D., & Sato, A. "The possible role of female sex hormones in milk from pregnant cows in the development of cancers." *Medical Hypotheses* 65.6 (2005): 1028–1037.
- Allen, N. E., et al. "A prospective study of dietary dairy intake and prostate cancer risk." *American Journal of Clinical Nutrition* 87.2 (2008): 497–505.
- Abelow, B. J., Holford, T. R., & Insogna, K. L. "Cross-cultural association between dietary animal protein and hip fracture: a hypothesis." *Calcified Tissue International* 50 (1992): 14–18.
- Uribarri, J., et al. "Advanced glycation end products in foods and a practical guide to their reduction in the diet." *Journal of the American Dietetic Association* 110.6 (2010): 911–916.
- Dethlefsen, C., Højfeldt, G., & Hojman, P. "The role of intratumoral and systemic IL-6 in breast cancer." *Breast Cancer Research and Treatment* 138.3 (2013): 657–664.
- Shaw, R. J. "AMPK signaling: maintaining energy homeostasis at the crossroads of metabolism and cancer." *Cell* 161.3 (2015): 456–470.
- Saxton, R. A., & Sabatini, D. M. "mTOR signaling in growth, metabolism, and disease." *Cell* 168.6 (2017): 960–976.
- Warburg, O. *The Metabolism of Tumours*. Richard R. Smith, 1931.
Giovannucci, E., et al. "Dairy products, calcium, and prostate cancer risk." *Cancer Epidemiology, Biomarkers & Prevention* 15.2 (2006): 203–210.
- Levine, M. E., et al. "Low protein intake is associated with a major reduction in IGF-1, cancer, and overall mortality in the 65 and younger but not older population." *Cell Metabolism* 19.3 (2014): 407–417.

Chapter 5

- Campbell, T. Colin, and Thomas M. Campbell II. *The China Study*. BenBella Books, 2006.
- Qin, L. Q., et al. "Milk consumption and circulating insulin-like growth factor-I level: a systematic literature review." *European Journal of Clinical Nutrition* 64.12 (2010): 1331–1339.

• Parodi, P. W. "A role for milk proteins and their peptides in cancer prevention and treatment." *Current Pharmaceutical Design* 13.8 (2007): 813–828.

• Ganmaa, Davaasambuu, and Akiko Sato. "The possible role of female sex hormones in milk from pregnant cows in the development of breast, ovarian and corpus uteri cancers." *Medical Hypotheses* 65.6 (2005): 1028–1037.

• Gill, H. S., and K. J. Cross. "Bovine milk peptides and mucosal immunity." *International Dairy Journal* 10.1-2 (2000): 69–78.

• Gomariz, M. J., et al. "Inflammatory cytokines, LPS and histamine: molecular and cellular aspects in mucosal immunity." *Allergologia et Immunopathologia* 27.2 (1999): 72–79.

• Nedergaard, Maiken, et al. "The glymphatic system (GLS): A waste clearance system in the brain." *Science* 340.6140 (2013): 1529–1531.

Chapter 6

• Ozturk, G., et al. "Effects of industrial heat treatments on the kinetics of xanthine oxidase in milk." *NPJ Science of Food*, 3 (2019): 13. nature.com

• Zikakis, J.P. "Activity of Xanthine Oxidase in Dairy Products." *Journal of Dairy Science*, 63.7 (1980): 1251-1256. journalofdairyscience.org

• Ho, C.Y., Clifford, A.J., Swenerton, H. "Homogenized bovine milk xanthine oxidase: a critique of the hypothesis relating to plasmalogen depletion and cardiovascular disease." *American Journal of Clinical Nutrition*, 38.2 (1983): 327-332. scholarworks.moreheadstate.edu

• Praepanitchai, O.-A. "The influence of pasteurization temperatures, homogenization pressures and storage duration at 4 °C on activity of milk xanthine oxidase." Master's thesis, University of Tennessee, 1977. trace.tennessee.edu

• "On the supposed influence of milk homogenization on the risk of CVD, diabetes and allergy." *British Journal of Nutrition*, 97.4 (2007): 598-610. Cambridge University Press & Assessment

• "Raw Milk Misconceptions and the Danger of Raw Milk Consumption." United States Food & Drug Administration. U.S. Food and Drug Administration

Chapter 7

• Frassetto, L. A., et al. "Diet, evolution and aging—the pathophysiologic effects of the post-agricultural inversion of the potassium-to-sodium and base-to-chloride ratios in the human diet." *European Journal of Nutrition* 40.5 (2001): 200–213.

• Sellmeyer, D. E., et al. "A high ratio of dietary animal to vegetable protein increases the rate of bone loss and the risk of fracture in postmenopausal women." *American Journal of Clinical Nutrition* 77.2 (2003): 504–511.

• Warburg, Otto. *The Metabolism of Tumours*. Richard R. Smith, 1931.

• Cani, Patrice D., et al. "Metabolic endotoxemia initiates obesity and insulin resistance." *Diabetes* 56.7 (2007): 1761–1772.

• Lerner, Aaron, and Torsten Matthias. "Changes in intestinal tight junction permeability associated with industrial food additives." *Autoimmunity Reviews* 14.6 (2015): 479–489.

• Fasano, Alessio. "Zonulin and its regulation of intestinal barrier function: the biological door to inflammation, autoimmunity, and cancer." *Physiological Reviews* 91.1 (2011): 151–175.

• Capuron, Lucile, and Andrew H. Miller. "Immune system to brain signaling: neuropsychopharmacological implications." *Pharmacology & Therapeutics* 130.2 (2011): 226–238.

• Melnik, Bodo C. "Milk—a nutrient system of mammalian evolution promoting mTORC1-dependent translation." *International Journal of Molecular Sciences* 16.8 (2015): 17048–17087.

Chapter 8

• Boden, G., et al. "Effects of free fatty acids on glucose uptake and utilization in humans." *Journal of Clinical Investigation* 93.6 (1994): 2438–2446.

• Itani, S. I., et al. "Lipid-induced insulin resistance in human muscle is associated with changes in diacylglycerol, protein kinase C, and IkB-α." *Diabetes* 51 (2002): 2005–2011.

• Melnik, B. C. "Milk—A nutrient system of mammalian evolution promoting mTORC1-dependent translation." *International Journal of Molecular Sciences* 16 (2015): 17048–17087.

• Calder, P. C. "Polyunsaturated fatty acids and inflammatory processes: new twists in an old tale." *Biochimie* 91.6 (2009): 791–795.

Summers, S. A. "Ceramides in insulin resistance and lipotoxicity." *Progress in Lipid Research* 45.1 (2006): 42–72.

• Aune, D., et al. "Dairy products and the risk of type 2 diabetes: a systematic review and dose-response meta-analysis." *American Journal of Clinical Nutrition* 98.4 (2013): 1066–1083.

• Choi, H. K., et al. "Dairy consumption and risk of type 2 diabetes in men: a prospective study." *Archives of Internal Medicine* 165.9 (2005): 997–1003.

• Ganmaa, D., & Sato, A. "The possible role of female sex hormones in milk from pregnant cows in the development of cancers and hormonal disorders." *Medical Hypotheses* 65.6 (2005): 1028–1037.

• Barnard, N. D., et al. "A low-fat vegan diet improves glycemic control and cardiovascular risk factors in a randomized clinical trial in individuals with type 2 diabetes." *Diabetes Care* 29.8 (2006): 1777–1783.

Chapter 9:

• Akimoto, Takashi, et al. "Role of Phospholipase A2 in Inflammation and Cellular Signaling." *Progress in Lipid Research*, vol. 48, no. 1, 2009, pp. 27–40.

• Bagga, Deepak, et al. "Dietary Modulation of the Omega-6/Omega-3 Ratio and Eicosanoid Production." *Proceedings of the National Academy of Sciences*, vol. 99, no. 9, 2002, pp. 6052–6056.

• Bannenberg, Gary L., and Charles N. Serhan. "Specialized Pro-Resolving Lipid Mediators in Inflammation." *Journal of Clinical Investigation*, vol. 116, no. 10, 2006, pp. 2517–2525.

• Basak, Subrata, et al. "Arachidonic Acid Pathways and Their Role in Inflammation." *International Journal of Inflammation*, vol. 2010, 2010, Article ID 809042.

• Bengtsson, Anne M., et al. "Dietary Intake of Dairy Fat Increases Plasma Arachidonic Acid." *Lipids*, vol. 47, 2012, pp. 381–389.

• Calder, Philip C. "The Relationship Between the Arachidonic Acid:EPA Ratio and Inflammation." *International Journal of Clinical Practice*, vol. 71, 2017, e12920.

• Calder, Philip C. "Polyunsaturated Fatty Acids, Inflammation, and Immunity." *Nutrition*, vol. 16, no. 7–8, 2000, pp. 688–703.

• Caughey, Gillian E., et al. "High Consumption of Omega-6 Polyunsaturated Fatty Acids Increases Inflammatory Markers." *American Journal of Clinical Nutrition*, vol. 87, no. 4, 2008, pp. 957–966.

• Chiurchiù, Valerio, and Mauro Maccarrone. "Arachidonic Acid Pathways and the Nervous System." *Trends in Neurosciences*, vol. 41, no. 8, 2018, pp. 612–627.

• Dantzer, Robert, et al. "From Inflammation to Sickness and Depression: When the Immune System Subjugates the Brain." *Nature Reviews Neuroscience*, vol. 9, 2008, pp. 46–56.

• Engström, Anna M. R., et al. "Dairy Consumption Increases the Arachidonic Acid Content of Immune Cell Phospholipids." *British Journal of Nutrition*, vol. 106, no. 6, 2011, pp. 825–832.

• Ferreira, Sérgio H., and John R. Vane. "Prostaglandins: Their Role in Pain and Inflammation." *Nature*, vol. 240, 1972, pp. 200–203.

• Funk, Colin D. "Prostaglandins and Leukotrienes: Advances in Eicosanoid Biology." *Science*, vol. 294, no. 5548, 2001, pp. 1871–1875.

• Ginty, Annie T., et al. "Milk Fat Intake and Systemic Inflammation." *Journal of Nutrition & Metabolism*, vol. 2013, 2013, Article ID 490507.

• Hansen, Harald S., et al. "Arachidonic Acid and Endothelial Function." *American Journal of Clinical Nutrition*, vol. 71, no. 1, 2000, pp. 318–324.

• Harizi, Halima, and Nabil Gualde. "Eicosanoids: Cross-Talk Between the Immune and Nervous Systems." *Neuroscience*, vol. 138, no. 3, 2006, pp. 957–967.

• Hinz, Burkhard, et al. "Prostaglandins as Modulators of Neuronal Function." *Pharmacology & Therapeutics*, vol. 124, no. 3, 2009, pp. 215–241.

• Hjorth, Mads, et al. "Dairy Fat Intake Alters Plasma Fatty Acid Composition and Inflammatory Markers." *European Journal of Clinical Nutrition*, vol. 68, no. 9, 2014, pp. 1034–1040.

• Hurst, Simon M., et al. "Quinolinic Acid, Neuroinflammation, and NMDA Receptor Toxicity." *Journal of Neuroinflammation*, vol. 5, 2008, 14.

• Kelley, D. S., and Barry D. Temple. "Modulation of Humoral Immunity by Dietary Fatty Acids." *Journal of Nutrition*, vol. 131, no. 9, 2001, pp. 2568–2573.

• Kiecolt-Glaser, Janice K., et al. "Omega-6 Fatty Acids and Inflammation-Driven Depression." *Brain, Behavior, and Immunity*, vol. 25, no. 6, 2011, pp. 1119–1126.

• Kohyama, Noriko, et al. "Eicosanoids and Endocrine Regulation." *Prostaglandins & Other Lipid Mediators*, vol. 123, 2016, pp. 13–25.

• Liu, Yizhe, et al. "Cytokine-Induced Activation of Indoleamine-2,3-Dioxygenase and Tryptophan Depletion." *Psychoneuroendocrinology*, vol. 36, no. 9, 2011, pp. 1391–1398.

• Martín, Carlos R., et al. "Dairy-Derived Hormones and Human Endocrine Disruption." *Journal of Endocrinology*, vol. 232, 2017, pp. R67–R80.

• Mendonça, Raquel, et al. "Arachidonic Acid Overload and Mitochondrial Dysfunction." *Biochimica et Biophysica Acta (BBA) – Molecular Cell Research*, vol. 1864, no. 12, 2017, pp. 2019–2032.

• Nath, Neetu, et al. "Inflammation-Driven IDO Pathway: Link Between Mood and Immunity." *Journal of Neurochemistry*, vol. 120, no. 6, 2012, pp. 851–861.

• Nathan, Carl. "Points of Control in Inflammation." *Nature*, vol. 420, 2002, pp. 846–852.

• Okuyama, Hiroshi, et al. "Excess Omega-6 Fatty Acids and Cardiovascular Disease." *Biomedicine & Pharmacotherapy*, vol. 70, 2015, pp. 417–421.

• Russo, George L. "Dietary N-6 Polyunsaturated Fatty Acids and Pro-Inflammatory Eicosanoids." *Nutrition and Cancer*, vol. 61, no. 5, 2009, pp. 573–583.

• Serhan, Charles N., et al. "Resolvins, Protectins, and the End of Inflammation." *Journal of Experimental Medicine*, vol. 206, no. 1, 2009, pp. 15–23.

• Simopoulos, Artemis P. "The Importance of the Omega-6/Omega-3 Ratio in Health." *Experimental Biology and Medicine*, vol. 233, no. 6, 2008, pp. 674–688.

• Sordillo, Lorraine M., and Shaun P. Raphael. "Inflammatory Mediators in Dairy Fat." *Journal of Dairy Science*, vol. 96, no. 7, 2013, pp. 3927–3935.

• Vane, John R., and Louis J. Kunkel. "Cyclooxygenase Pathways and Prostaglandins." *Annual Review of Biochemistry*, vol. 79, 2010, pp. 461–480.

• Wang, Qing, et al. "Endothelial Dysfunction Induced by Arachidonic Acid Metabolites." *American Journal of Physiology–Heart and Circulatory Physiology*, vol. 310, 2016, pp. H1–H10.

• Yang, Rui, et al. "Excess Omega-6 Fatty Acids and Neuroinflammation." *Molecular Psychiatry*, vol. 26, 2021, pp. 143–154.

Chapter 10

• Ganmaa, D., & Sato, A. "The possible role of female sex hormones in milk from pregnant cows in the development of breast, ovarian and corpus uteri cancers." *Medical Hypotheses* 65 (2005): 1028–1037.

• Maruyama, K., et al. "Exposure to exogenous estrogen through intake of commercial milk produced from pregnant cows." *Pediatric International* 52 (2010): 33–38.

• Peeters, P. H. M., et al. "Breast cancer risk associated with dairy consumption." *Journal of the National Cancer Institute* 86 (1994): 936–942.

• Akingbemi, B. T. "Estrogen regulation of testicular function." *Reproductive Biology and Endocrinology* 3 (2005): 51.

• Jelen, P., & Liptáková, D. "Cortisol levels in milk of dairy cows under stress." *Czech Journal of Animal Science* 53 (2008): 436–441.

• Giovannucci, E., et al. "Milk and dairy foods, IGF-1 and prostate cancer risk." *Cancer Epidemiology Biomarkers & Prevention* 12 (2003): 1081–1085.

• Melnik, B. C. "Milk signaling through mTORC1: a mechanism explaining common diseases of civilization." *Nutrients* 5 (2013): 1034–1061.

• Tomaszewska, E., et al. "Placental transfer of steroid hormones and milk-derived estrogens." *Journal of Endocrinology* 232 (2017): R81–R93.

• Virtanen, S. M., et al. "Cow's milk consumption in infancy and development of type 1 diabetes mellitus." *Diabetologia* 37 (1994): 381–387.

• Kolodziej, E. P., et al. "Steroid hormones, dairy effluent, and aquatic feminization." *Environmental Science & Technology* 37 (2003): 1748–1753.

• Barnard, N. D., et al. "A low-fat vegan diet improves hormonal profiles and menstrual pain." *European Journal of Clinical Nutrition* 69 (2015): 1228–1233.

Chapter 11

• Rios-Covian, D. et al. "Intestinal short-chain fatty acids and their link with diet and human health." *Frontiers in Microbiology* 7 (2016): 185.

• Bhat, M. I., & Kapila, R. "Cow milk casein-derived bioactive peptides: impact on human health." *Comprehensive Reviews in Food Science and Food Safety* 16 (2017): 1183–1198.

• Cani, P. D. et al. "Metabolic endotoxemia initiates obesity and insulin resistance." *Diabetes* 56 (2007): 1761–1772.

• Erridge, C. et al. "A high-fat meal induces low-grade endotoxemia." *American Journal of Clinical Nutrition* 86 (2007): 1286–1292.

• Cryan, J. F., & Dinan, T. G. "Mind-altering microorganisms: the impact of the gut microbiota on brain and behavior." *Nature Reviews Neuroscience* 13 (2012): 701–712.

• Dantzer, R. et al. "From inflammation to sickness and depression." *Nature Reviews Neuroscience* 9 (2008): 46–56.

• Lerner, A., & Matthias, T. "Changes in intestinal tight-junction permeability associated with food additives and autoimmunity." *Autoimmunity Reviews* 14 (2015): 479–489.

• Oliver, S. P. et al. "Foodborne pathogens in milk and the dairy farm environment." *Foodborne Pathogens and Disease* 6 (2009): 681–697.

• David, L. A. et al. "Diet rapidly and reproducibly alters the human gut microbiome." *Nature* 505 (2014): 559–563.

Chapter 12

• Abelow, B. J., Holford, T. R., & Insogna, K. L. "Cross-cultural association between dietary animal protein and hip fracture: a hypothesis." *Calcified Tissue International* 50 (1992): 14–18.

• Feskanich, D., et al. "Milk, dietary calcium, and bone fractures in women: a 12-year prospective study." *American Journal of Public Health* 87 (1997): 992–997.

• Nordin, B. E. C. "Calcium and osteoporosis." *Nutrition* 13 (1997): 664–686.

• Barzel, U. S., & Massey, L. K. "Excess dietary protein can adversely affect bone." *Journal of Nutrition* 128 (1998): 1051–1053.

• Kerstetter, J. E., et al. "The effect of dietary protein on calcium metabolism and bone health." *Current Opinion in Lipidology* 14 (2003): 45–52.

• Calvo, M. S., & Uribarri, J. "Contributions to total phosphorus intake: all sources considered." *Seminars in Dialysis* 26 (2013): 54–61.

• Melnik, B. C. "Milk signaling through mTORC1: a mechanism explaining common diseases of civilization." *Nutrients* 5 (2013): 1034–1061.

• Rennenberg, R. J. M. W., et al. "Calcium phosphate calcification in arterial walls." *Atherosclerosis* 207 (2009): 408–423.

• Nestle, M. *Food Politics: How the Food Industry Influences Nutrition and Health.* University of California Press, 2007.

• Lanou, A. J., et al. "Calcium, dairy products, and bone health in children and young adults: a reevaluation of the evidence." *Pediatrics* 115 (2005): 736–743.

• U.S. Department of Health & Human Services. *Bone Health and Osteoporosis: A Report of the Surgeon General.* 2004.

Chapter 13

• Ríos-Covián, D. et al. "Intestinal short-chain fatty acids and their link with diet and human health." *Frontiers in Microbiology* 7 (2016): 185.

• David, L. A. et al. "Diet rapidly and reproducibly alters the human gut microbiome." *Nature* 505 (2014): 559–563.

• Higdon, J. V., & Delage, B. "Cruciferous vegetables and human health." *Pharmacological Research* 55 (2007): 224–236.

• Pizzorno, J., et al. *Textbook of Natural Medicine.* 5th ed., Elsevier, 2020.

• Pollack, G. H. *The Fourth Phase of Water: Beyond Solid, Liquid, and Vapor.* Ebner and Sons, 2013.

• Melnik, B. C. "Milk—a nutrient system of mammalian evolution promoting mTORC1-dependent translation." *International Journal of Molecular Sciences* 16 (2015): 17048–17087.

• Cani, P. D., & Delzenne, N. M. "The role of the gut microbiota in energy metabolism and metabolic disease." *Current Pharmaceutical Design* 15 (2009): 1546–1558.

www.ingramcontent.com/pod-product-compliance
Lightning Source LLC
Chambersburg PA
CBHW081409270326
41931CB00016B/3423